UNRAVELLING THE SIGNS

LIVING WITH A DEAF SCHIZOPHRENIC BROTHER

SYLVIA KENNETH

First published in 2014 by
Action Deafness Books

Copyright © 2014 Action Deafness Books

A CIP Catalogue of this book is available from
the British Library

ISBN: 978-0-9570822-1-2

Cover designed by
Euan Carter
(www.euancarter.com)

Original photograph copyright Kwest

Typeset by
www.chandlerbookdesign.co.uk

Printed in Great Britain by
Berforts Information Press,
Stevenage, Hertfordshire

CONTENTS

Soon after Philip's death I began to reminisce about the past, thinking, reflecting. Many memories came flooding back: the time we spent together, holidays and weekends by the seaside, the fun we had together. The life he'd had haunted me for days. I also felt a dreadful remorse that I'd not found a way to step in when his illness became a problem. The guilt has racked me. Should I have helped Philip more with his mental state? Should I have sought professional help? Should I have asked people who'd had experience of dealing with mental health? Had we done enough to help Philip? I've always been one to mind my own business unless I am seriously asked to help, but I now wonder if that was enough to unravel the signs? I guess we will never know...

Foreword

Consultant Psychiatrist Dr Helen Miller

'Life is a grand adventure - or it is nothing'
Helen Keller

I work with Sylvia in a mental health hospital for Deaf people based in London that covers the southern third of England. We have worked together for over 10 years now; initially Sylvia was a health care assistant and now she is a charge nurse on our in-patient unit. I am a consultant psychiatrist who has specialised in working with Deaf adults who predominantly use British Sign Language.

I am very grateful to Sylvia for her courage and honesty in sharing with us the story of her brother's life and his battle with schizophrenia. This is the only biography I have come across about a Deaf person with schizophrenia and I will be recommending it to all my patients and their families.

She writes beautifully and her own remarkable personality and strength shines through the pages of this book. She shares with us stories from her family's history and from her childhood growing up in London, one of three Deaf and three hearing siblings. Her older brother who is Deaf developed schizophrenia in his late teens and the family embarked on a journey of loss and adjustment, as the illness took hold and his personality and behaviour deteriorated.

Schizophrenia is a very common illness and yet sufferers and their families are often left feeling confused by what is happening and isolated, judged and rejected by society. In my experience, Deafness exacerbates the problems schizophrenia causes. One of the reasons for this is the lack of accounts in the literature of Deaf people with serious mental illness. Deaf people have to rely on literature written by hearing people that never entirely matches their own experiences.

This book closes that gap and takes us a step towards reducing the isolation and confusion Deaf people with schizophrenia and their families suffer. To quote the journalist Rebecca Atkinson, who herself is Deaf and losing her sight:

'Through times of desperate isolation I have learned the painful lesson that denial comes with a heavy price to mental health, and resistance only results in failure. In other words, if you don't admit it, you start to feel you're losing the plot'.

Helen Miller

This book is dedicated to my
mother and father who have tirelessly
kept the family together throughout
the difficult years.

Edna – (1921-2008)

Frank – (1914-1994)

In loving memory of my brothers Ian
(1945-2008) and Philip (1954-1999).

"There are three different rules for reading, for thinking, and for talking. Writing blends all three of them."

Mason Cooley, 1993

Acknowledgements

I wish to express my sincere thanks to:

Members of the Kenneth family for helping collate our family history - Ian (deceased October 2008), Lillian, Alan, Jackie, Richard and Paul.

Team Leader Sonia Waring, Psychologist Lyn Galbraith, and Social Worker Jackie Biss, all at Rampton Hospital, for encouraging me to write this book.

My old school friends, Yvonne Clarke, Susan Gondor and Steven Cannadine for great memories of schooldays gone by!

Jackie McKay for her support and letting me stay with her for a couple of days when going through family crisis.

Elvire Roberts for giving me legal advice and lots of support.

Hannah Cobb for being there for me when I went through difficult times, and giving me inspirational stories of her life. We became emotionally stronger when we shared deep thoughts.

Paula Cox for sharing family experiences on schizophrenia.

Judith Newsome for being my travelling companion when we went backpacking to India and Nepal for five months.

Maggie Trent for tips on journalism and book writing.

BSL Interpreters Jill Robinson, Fleur Shaddick, Darrel Firth and Dionne Deans for checking my English and grammar.

Stephanie Cobb, Martin Ring, Donna Lewin, Rob Chalk, Siddika Kardi, Esther Thomas and Justina Mills for assisting me with queries relating to publishing of this book.

Jacqui Beckford for tips on publishing and books.

Tavis King for advice on books and scanning photographs.

Nicola Roeder, Frances Ridgewell, Sandra Mansfield, Lana Senchal and Anne Wheeler for being my lifelong friends.

My wider friends within the Deaf community who have shared their stories and experiences.

Lastly, I would also like to thank Action Deafness for their advice and support throughout the process - for the editing, proofreading, layout, publishing and for basically making the book happen!

All these people have helped me make this book possible and for that I am eternally grateful.

Introduction

The thought of writing a book about schizophrenia never occurred to me until a July day in 2008. On the day in question, Psychologist Lyn Galbraith, student Social Worker Jackie Biss, and myself were in the nurses' office discussing a certain patient who, having a personality disorder, thought he was famous and wished to be a writer. It was then that we talked about writing books and Lyn casually mentioned that she had already written a volume on children and psychology, titled *Theory of Mind*. I made a fleeting remark about wanting to write about my own experiences of living with a Deaf schizophrenic brother. Lyn couldn't contain herself and was full of encouragement, 'Write, write!' she gasped. 'Get your ideas down and get it together!' She was full of enthusiasm and it was this that got me started. Jackie too was hugely supportive and she chipped in with the title '*Living with a Deaf Schizophrenic Brother*'. So that's how my dream of writing this difficult story began.

This work has taken time to compile as over the years my memories of family life have faded and I am consequently reliant on memory jogs and flashbacks. As these can and do happen anywhere, whether I am on a train, bus, driving a car, going shopping, talking with somebody or even sound asleep, I had to scribble down notes on pieces of paper to help me to hold on to each fleeting memory! I took to carrying a small notebook, which accompanied me everywhere and I found this extremely useful. Over the years and especially in recent months, distant memories have been coming to the fore. Although I thought these vivid images would be easy to recall at a later date, they quickly faded back into the past. But with my notebook, I was able to capture them and note them down.

From the moment I decided to write this story, I scribbled every thought and recollection onto my little pad. On many occasions, I woke in the middle of the night, switched on the lamp, jotted down a few scrambled words and promptly went back to sleep. My dreams are always different and my recollections of past events come back in varying forms. Occasionally, I have the odd bad dream as most people do, but each memory I have is unique and so I try to reflect upon and value each of them as I write them down.

Once you start to carry a notebook, you realise how important it is. I wonder sometimes whether other writers experience these thoughts at all times of the day and I wonder how many of them share their thoughts with notebooks of blank pages! Sometimes when you have a pen or pencil ready to scribble down, the memory can vanish or you become lost while trying to figure out what to write. I talked about this experience with my friends and they agreed that it can happen wherever you are, that you get a memory jog or flashback from the past in the most peculiar places. I am sure many other writers would agree with me that they carry scraps of paper or a notepad for this purpose!

At first I was reluctant to write this book, because I was afraid of criticism from the public and from those families that have experienced schizophrenia. I was afraid of the reaction in my workplace and the possibility that some healthcare professionals would not agree with what I write. Despite this fear, I also understood that everyone has differing views and perspectives on mental health and schizophrenia. I suspect that a lot of parents who have not had any experience of mental illness or drug addiction might find some parts hard to read and that this might make it hard for them to relate to my family. But people need to know that mental illness does happen to families like ours and, indeed, I am sure there are many ordinary families who will relate to my story. I would like to share my experiences in the hope that many more people will have a better understanding of mental health issues and be inspired by the strength that surrounds them.

I am aware that my story will explore a very sensitive issue but as Lyn said, my story is in one respect very unique - it is not only the experience of having a schizophrenic brother, but it is also the experience of us both being born profoundly Deaf. Sharing that cultural identity together, having a common ground and then going through the diagnosis of schizophrenia has made me realise what it means to have a Deaf schizophrenic brother. Lyn challenged me to search to see if I could find a similar story to mine in print or on the internet - she was absolutely right, I could find no account of a Deaf family experiencing the challenge of schizophrenia. So here I am, trying my determined best to do this story justice. This book is based upon the memories of my own life experience and within those memories are painful episodes of disruption and despair. My brother's mental illness affected my family and me in many ways, but I feel I am now ready to share them.

Unravelling the Signs: Living with a Deaf Schizophrenic Brother is divided into two parts. The first part is called *The Early Years* which provides an insight into my family background with various childhood memories and stories. The second part is called *How My Brother Developed Schizophrenia* and it reveals the effect my brother, and schizophrenia, had on my family and the people we knew.

I am fortunate that members of my family have agreed and encouraged me to write this book and they have supported me all the way. I am one of three siblings who are congenitally, genetically Deaf, and who have three other brothers, who are what we call in the Deaf community 'hearing'. One of my Deaf siblings had schizophrenia and so my childhood experience was shaped by exposure to someone who was mentally ill. My family believe that this account will benefit other people and that, yes, there may be criticism of what I have written. But I'm ready for that, given that what I have written is as I lived it, true to my memory. I have not exaggerated or whitewashed anything. Although I have had difficult times, I hold no hard feelings against my family or childhood, and I continue to love my family as always and forever.

I try not to describe myself as 'a writer' in this book - writing for me is not a career activity but rather an outlet for expression. Reflecting on how I started to write this story, I can see what a powerful impact it has made on me. Even as I continue to write this work, I'm repeatedly going back to the beginning to revisit and rewrite some of the passages.

I remember about 15 years ago, I went to a psychic fair held in the local library with two of my friends. As I was walking along I noticed a clairvoyant talking to a customer and reading her hands; I walked past but I had a strong urge to meet the clairvoyant; I felt there was a magnetism drawing me towards this lady. I'm not a believer in such things so I tried to ignore it, but I was drawn back to her. So I waited in the queue and when my turn came, I sat down with her and she welcomed me with a warming, expectant smile. The clairvoyant asked if it was my first time and I confirmed that this was the case. I was puzzled and wondered, 'How did she know that? She does not even know me, so how can she read my mind?' The clairvoyant asked my friend to interpret for me, rubbing my white-gold ring whilst holding my hand, and poured out details of my past, present and future. She reflected on Dad being ill and my brother who had a sad life. But to me, the most important thing she said was, 'You're a creative writer: use this talent, make use of it!' At the time I thought it was nonsense and that I was hopeless at writing, but now I agree! I believe that when you have the urge to write then you must follow your instincts; write, get it down, express yourself...

Many, many people have the ability to write and express themselves in books, articles or even newspapers. Of course, it is a matter of what and when to write, finding the right place and time - but anyone can write a book! It amazes me when I go to a bookshop and see shelf upon shelf of books written by so many different people. I am certain these books are eye-openers for those that settle down to read them - both an illumination and education. It is such a wonderful feeling to read, I can't encourage you enough - go on, enjoy, read, learn and perhaps write yourself!

PART ONE

The Early Years and Family History

1

My Father

My dad, Frank Kenneth, was a Scotsman born in the fishing village of Arbroath in 1914. He was the seventh of eight children with four sisters and three brothers: Nellie, Agnes, Esther, Jean, George junior, James and Logie. Dad's parents had lived in Arbroath for all their lives. Of strict Presbyterian stock, the Kenneth family regularly attended the Church of Scotland and were devoted to their faith.

The name Kenneth originated from the clan of the Mackenzies, the crest of the Mackenzie's armorial bearings being a stag's head and horns. It is said that they were assumed in consequence of Kenneth, the ancestor of the family, having rescued the King of Scotland from an infuriated stag which he had wounded 'in gratitude for his assistance'. Historical writings show that 'the king gave him a grant of the castle and lands of Castle Donnan, and thus laid the foundation of the family and clan Mackenneth or Mackenzie'1. From the stag's head on their coat of arms the term 'Caberfae' (the deer's head) was adopted for the chiefs.

---

1 Taken from www.electricscotland.com/webclans/m/mackenz

In generations before, Dad's family had lived hard lives on the east coast, eking out livelihoods as fishermen working the dangerous Scottish waters. However, my grandfather, George senior, was a master baker and his reputation in Arbroath was second to none. There was never a finer baker than George Kenneth!

Dad always boasted about his surname and how proud he was of his regal Scots ancestry. When I was young, I was unsure whether these stories were true but through reading numerous great tomes on Scottish history, I later realised the tales were indeed true! When I immersed myself in these volumes, I found it interesting to learn of Scottish culture, tradition and attitudes; their roots traced back to distant Celtic tribal systems. The clans (families) fought ferociously over the years for their rights, such that today, each clan is proud of territorial distinctions, customs and, of course, their tartans, worn today with pride!

The Kenneth family lived in a corner house which stood just a short distance from Arbroath's cobbled harbour. With a population today of some 23,000, Arbroath is situated in the county of Angus, east central Scotland, on the North Sea and at the mouth of the Brothock River. It is famous for its fabulous 'smokies', haddock fillets that have been smoked over oak hardwood until they take on a beautiful burnished-gold colour and a full, smoky flavour.

Stories of old have it that the smokie was first created when a haddock was discovered in the embers of a burning cottage in Arbroath. The haddock - which was charred from the fire - was sampled by some fishermen who found it to be delicious. Since then the smoked fish has become a tradition that is still going strong. Today Arbroath smokies are exported all over the world and if you are holidaying in or around Arbroath, you just need to follow the warm oaky smell to discover the backstreet smokehouses.

I seem to recall that Dad regularly had kippers for Sunday breakfast along with rough-hewn bread and butter, with which he wiped the plate clean. He used to take out the tiny bones one by one whilst he ate. It's funny but when I think of him patiently eating his Sunday breakfast, I can still recall that distinctive smell. Not only did Dad love his kippers but also haggis accompanied by 'tatties and neeps' (potatoes and turnips). He adored this traditional fare made from a delectable mixture of pig's offal and oats, as is famously eaten every Burns' night on the 31st January. A date surely permanently etched in every Scotsman's calendar!?

George senior died of pneumonia when Dad was only 12 years old. His shocked mother had to keep eight children on a widow's benefit (there was no National Health Service in those days, during the early 1920s). This was a struggle for her and she died shortly afterwards leaving Dad's elder sister Nellie, and her husband, Stanley senior, to look after the family.

When Dad turned 15 years of age, he decided to leave Arbroath as he wanted to travel. He joined a band of Romanies (some people refer to them as Gypsies) and travelled all across Scotland. Dad must have been so brave to join this band at his young age, but he wanted to embark on a new life journey, despite it taking him far away from his family back in Arbroath.

The work of the Romany in those days was varied but hard. It was mainly farm work - hunting, poaching, wood-carving, metalwork, patching and mending, the grinding of knives, shears, scythes, axes and more. I remember Dad told me a story of how he had worked on one particular farm where he was in an abattoir, slaughtering livestock. With great remorse, he described to me how electric guns were used to kill cows, the stun bolt being fired at their temples. He asked me to forgive him for his part in these killings, but I understood that he had to work to live and this was what was expected of him. Dad later admitted that he hated that job and that he couldn't wait to leave. He got away as soon as he could after just a year.

One day, when the travellers were moving along, Dad was a passenger in a Romany bowtop wagon, sitting alongside his companion who was mindfully steering the horse. Suddenly, out of nowhere, a coal lorry hurtled down at a crossroads and crashed into them. In the resultant, awful collision, Dad was seriously injured with compound fractures to his right leg and he had to endure a lengthy stay in Perth Infirmary Hospital. He spent weeks in hospital where a large silver metal plate was inserted in his thigh and he had to have 40 stitches across the side of his leg. He received a large compensation payment for his injuries which was collected by his brother-in-law, Stanley, who brought him back home. In later years, Dad told us that the compensation money was given to his brothers, George junior and James, to help them set up a bakery business, all of which sought to capitalise upon grandfather's success and influence as a master baker. Dad was promised and assured that the money would be returned - but it was never forthcoming and he was left feeling most bitter. Yet the bakery became very successful and went from strength to strength. At one point George junior and James made a beautiful wedding cake for the famous Scottish singer, Moira Anderson. She was a celebrated artist and appeared frequently at the London Palladium singing Scottish songs.

Whilst recovering in hospital, Dad was attended to by a nurse called Rosetta. She gently and dutifully attended to his needs and a little while later, a whirlwind romance occurred. Before long they married and bore two daughters, Kay Frances and Heather. But sadly, the marriage didn't last long and just before the beginning of the Second World War, Dad left his wife and daughters to move down south in the hope of finding a job and starting a new life. No one in the family quite knows why the marriage failed and Dad never talked about it, but I believe it was something to do with a family rift on Rosetta's side. I can only imagine that it must have been an impossible and painful decision for Dad to leave ... but perhaps the marriage was simply an unhappy one or perhaps he couldn't bear to be Romany any more. I don't know, but Dad moved south just as the clouds of war gathered over Europe.

During the Second World War, many men were called up to serve in the armed forces but Dad was rejected because of his leg injuries. He was classed as 'medically unfit'. When I was younger I pondered whether he had been a deserter who had deliberately shirked military service, but this wasn't the case. Even so, Dad made it clear after the war that he was glad he hadn't been in the army and that he certainly wouldn't have wanted to end up in the fighting!

Although nobody from the Kenneth family seems to remember Dad's training as an engineer, he was sent to London as a 'reserved occupation' engineer at a converted linoleum factory which became a torpedo factory in Staines. There was a rumour circulating amongst some members of the family that Dad had actually borrowed his brother Logie's engineer qualification papers to get the job, stating that Logie was Gaelic for Frank!

Dad and another man were the only men amongst the many hundreds of women working in the munitions factory. I can well imagine the women cracking jokes, teasing and goading their male counterparts. This is where my Dad met my mother. But whilst they fell in love and eventually started living together, they couldn't marry because even though Dad was separated, he was still legally married.

When my parents were courting during the early years of the war, they would often go for a romantic, night-time stroll along the River Thames - as many couples did and still do. On one occasion, they witnessed the London Blitz first hand as the fires caused by German bombing burned fiercely. My parents recalled the devastation visible across the city, and although the memory was marked with emotion and sadness, they could not help but describe the image of St Paul's Cathedral, stark against the backdrop of the red sky, a magnificent yet awful sight to behold amidst the terror and violence.

In Scotland, Dad's elder sister Nellie had two sons and a daughter: Malcolm, Stanley and Carolyn Fairweather. When my family went up to Scotland for holidays, Malcolm and Stanley used to tell us stories about Dad being a 'bit of a lad' and that he would get himself into all sorts of mischief. They said Uncle Frank was always in trouble and when just 15, he used to race with his friend on a motorbike along the narrow wall of the harbour! It was a crazy race and a highly dangerous thing to do, but they enjoyed the thrill of risking life and limb!

Dad learned to drive by 'borrowing' his brother James' car but this self-tutoring experience ended early when he crashed it into a petrol pump at the garage. Luckily for him and others, it did not burst into flames and so a catastrophic disaster was thankfully avoided. Dad's sister, Jean, told of a story that in his convertible car, Dad wore a college scarf and sunglasses whilst waving at people as he and a friend drove around town! Auntie Jean spotted them as they paraded along the main shopping street and she never let Dad forget this. It seems Dad was blessed with Clark Gable looks and that he was most popular with the ladies!

He was certainly a wit too. When we were up at Loch Ness, Dad would terrify us with stories of the large dinosaur-like monster living deep below. He talked of people having reported sightings of the monster and said that there were photographs to prove its existence. Dad said that if any of us went near the lake the monster would come up and snatch us away - believe it or not!

Dad was a self-taught craftsman and car mechanic. Highly skilled, he made lots of things from wood including a wall cabinet in the lounge, fitted kitchen cupboards, a doll's house and also a huge cocktail bar which I remember helping him construct. Without realising it, I learnt a lot of DIY skills from Dad and became proficient in the use of drills, screwdrivers, planes and even electrical wiring. A friend of Dad's asked him to design and build a seafood stall for the Robinson Crusoe pub in Green Lanes, Stoke Newington. This was designed to be a two-wheeled cart contraption that was strong enough to stand out in the parking area next to the pub, but could also be manoeuvred around. This was a tough assignment for Dad, but he got it done and the cart performed excellently! Dad also taught his sons about car engines and general mechanics. They subsequently all ended up fixing and reconditioning other people's cars. It was no wonder the driveway was always covered in patches of oil!

Dad was a conscientious man with a very strong work ethic, and he always brought home a regular wage. He was a fabulous father - a very proud man, always well-shaven, with a trimmed moustache. He polished his shoes on a Saturday morning and wore smart clothes to go to his usual haunt - the Robinson Crusoe pub and on other occasions, the Brownswood Park Tavern. He was known to his friends there as 'Frankie' or 'Jock' and after coming home he would take a good nap for two hours or so.

In the 1980's, Dad became a Freemason. The Freemasons are a secretive yet philanthropic organisation, well known for their charitable work and donations to those in need. Dad was inspired by his father who became a Scottish Master Mason in 1922. Members attending the Lodge refer to every member with brotherly respect and Dad was called 'Brother Frank'. My brothers Ian and Alan followed in Dad's footsteps and joined the Freemasons too but they only stayed until Dad's death. The Masonic Lodge was strictly for men only and I used to pester Dad as to the real reason he was a member. But he would remain tight-lipped and say nothing except that the organisation wasn't suitable for women. Yet there were benefits for my mother - when my Dad was busy at the Lodge, she was able to enjoy her spare time and do what she wanted.

There were one or two funny Freemason incidents that used to make us rock with laughter. One in particular stands out. We all went to a ladies' evening once at the Connaught Halls in London. Our best wear was the order of the night and Dad and my brothers were attired in traditional Scottish kilts whilst Mum, myself and my three sisters-in-law were in long gowns. As we entered the hall, we took the steps down into the lobby where Dad accidentally tripped up and promptly took a tumble! What he wore - or rather what he didn't wear - was revealed to all in its full glory!! Mum and my sister-in-laws were aghast but luckily I didn't notice as I was distracted by a passer-by. Let's just say that it was an evening that at the time we wanted to forget, but now, of course, we chuckle at the memory!

Dad was the focus of my life for much of my upbringing and people always called me a 'Daddy's girl'. Sadly, at the age of 77, he suffered from senile dementia and after three years, had to be admitted to a nursing home as my mother wasn't able to address his care needs. Dad stayed at the nursing home until his death five days before Christmas 1994. He died of pneumonia one week after a nasty fall which split his left eyebrow and needed several stitches. On the night he died, my mother's clock stopped at 3.30 am and mine at 3.45 am ... we've never been able to explain this strange coincidence. Needless to say, our Christmas celebration that year was a quiet, muted affair.

2

My Mother

My mum Edna was a true Londoner, born in Newington Green, north London. She was one of five, having two brothers, Reginald and Don, and two sisters, Connie and Gladys. Soon after she was born, her parents bought a house in Hedge Lane, Palmers Green, which was one of London's new pre-war urban developments.

Edna was a tall woman with dark hair and delicate features. Photographs of my mother as a youngster show her to have been very pretty and really quite the beauty amongst her sisters. Mum grew up to be a very jolly woman with a great sense of humour and a great belief in happiness. I always remember her words of wisdom that we should enjoy the good things in life and not be too materialistic. 'Money is the root of all evil', she would often say.

I was told by Mum's family that she was a brilliant swimmer and swam for one of London's top teams. Mum and her best friend Dolly were friends together in the team and they regularly met at the pool for practice sessions. She won a lot of medals and competed successfully against other teams, though she did not pursue a swimming career, choosing motherhood instead. She was a strong believer in family values, and sought to bring up her children to the best of her abilities.

In 1940, what with the men being away fighting the war, women moved in to take over jobs traditionally held by men. Some of these were really quite laborious and very hard work. So at the age of nineteen, Mum was sent to a torpedo factory with her two sisters Connie and Gladys. Her job was to stamp gyro settings on torpedo casings whilst her sister Gladys stamped on the Union Jack! Mum did not really talk much about the job or the war, saying that she found it all too depressing, though occasionally she would talk a little when the subject of the war came up at family gatherings.

I do remember she told us that air raid wardens wore steel helmets and used to go around the streets, making sure that people did not have any lights showing because they might guide in the German planes and show them where to bomb. All houses had to have blackout curtains made of thick black material to stop the light shining through. The warden would shout, 'Put that light out!' if they saw anyone with a light showing. She also distinctly remembered the sounds of Spitfires and Mosquitos roaring across the sky at night and of the huge American bombers that flew in daylight.

Mum's eldest brother Reginald died when he was just 20 years old due to tuberculosis. This was possibly contracted when he was a soldier posted overseas in the war. Mum, Connie, Gladys and Don would often talk about their dear brother whenever they met on family occasions. Reginald's fiancée Maud remained a family friend for years and was known to us as 'Auntie Maud'.

During the war, there were no televisions or computers and information was hard to come by. A lot of people listened to the radio for news, music, information or plays. Very few people had telephones and so information was passed by word of mouth. My Mum, her sisters and brothers would therefore often go home together after work to have tea together. Here, they would share news and gossip from the happenings of the day.

After the war, Mum worked part-time at the Maynards sweet factory which was just round from the private rented flat in Haringey, where we lived. Maynards was a well-known bakery which had become famous for making sweets such as wine gums, milk bottles and Brazil nuts coated in marzipan. Mum always brought home discounted sweets for us to savour. Hygiene was of paramount importance at Maynards and all the staff were provided with an apron and headwear that had to be worn every day. This was to ensure the production line was protected from germs.

In 1961, we moved to Bethune Road in Stoke Newington. Our street sat just on the corner of Grangecourt Road. The house was south-facing and we had no central heating, only a fireplace in the lounge. Going upstairs to the bedroom at night often felt like stepping into a freezer! On the coldest nights my parents would put extra woollen blankets and eiderdowns over us, but they would become so heavy we could hardly move.

Sometimes Paul and I would go down the bottom of Bethune Road to a tiny alleyway which led to the back of a huge coal yard. There was a small dented hole and we would steal pieces of coal and take them back to the coal bucket at home. My parents were not always aware of what we were doing even though the coal we 'acquired' was bigger and more roughly cut compared to the smaller pieces we already had in the bucket. Paul and I would sometimes get caught by Mum with our hands all black and dirty, but she would turn a blind eye and pretend nothing had happened. She told me in later years that she knew what was going on, but realised we meant well and were trying to keep the family warm. It was lovely though to have a roaring fire with the coals burning; it really heated the room up and I would watch the dancing of the blue flames for hours.

In the evenings, we would toast bread or crumpets on a long fork over the fire. Looking back, I can now see why there was a small dented hole at the back of the yard - it wasn't just us liberating the coal, there were others at it too!

As we were growing up and eating more food, Mum had to work more hours. She therefore took another part-time job as a cleaner for a Jewish family, the Rosenfelds, who lived just a few doors away from us. The Rosenfelds were very trusting of my mother and they gave her a lot of food as they knew we were hard up. They had a successful business which made handbags for the Jewish community and as with many other Jewish families at the time, all the extended family including siblings and children were involved in the business.

37a Bethune Road was a five-bedroom house with a kitchen and lounge. It was decided by my parents that one of the largest bedrooms would become a private lounge only to be used on special occasions. It was a grand room with two balconies. The house itself was on three storeys with a front door which led to an upstairs entrance. The house 37b was based on the ground floor and comprised two bedrooms, being adjacent to the right side of 37a. The first storey consisted of a bathroom, a small lounge and a kitchen. On the second storey, my parents' bedroom was located to the left and the next door opened to the private lounge. On the third storey was a long landing consisting of three bedrooms, all of which were situated on the right side. When we moved to this house, my twin brother and I had bunk beds in our parents' room. Ian and Alan shared the bedroom at the end of the third storey, whilst Richard and Philip had rooms further along.

The bunk bed was useful - Paul and I could communicate to each other if we wanted to. Sometimes in the middle of the night I would get his attention by raising both my feet and kicking the mattress above so we could talk. When it was really dark we would use torches to conduct our nocturnal conversing!

I can remember vividly Philip, Paul and I sliding down the banister from the third to the second landing rather than walking down the stairs. We would often get told off when sliding on the banister as we would crash onto the floor, annoying the neighbours below.

Mum spent a lot of time in the kitchen and she always had the radio on in the lounge. She loved to listen to music and would sometimes dance the jitterbug whilst pottering around in the small kitchen. We used to enjoy watching Mum dance as she created a happy, homely atmosphere. She loved her cigarettes too - John Player's Weights cigarettes which were simple filterless smokes, just tobacco wrapped in cigarette paper. She regularly left a lit one on top of the oven when busy with something else! Whenever Paul, Philip or I went to the local sweet shop, Mum would always ask us to buy a packet of five Weights cigarettes. She was always busy and sitting watching TV with her was a rare occurrence if ever. She always seemed to prefer to be in the kitchen.

Mum was constantly cooking for everybody, especially with six children and a husband to support. Things like peeling potatoes, slicing carrots and taking peas out of pods always remind me of her. In those days, we did not have a paring knife so we had to use an ordinary knife which was always difficult to master. Paul and I were taught how to peel a potato and slice it thinly so there was no waste. We always had a regular menu schedule for the week: mince stew or oxtail on Saturdays, roast beef or chicken on Sundays, steak and kidney pie on Mondays, liver and bacon with boiled potatoes on Tuesdays, cottage pie on Wednesdays, sausages, egg, chips and baked beans on Thursdays and of course, fish and chips from the local shop on Fridays! Thanks to my parents, we were never hungry. Many years later, I introduced Mum and Dad to the intricacies of a Chinese takeaway, but they were not at all impressed. Yet I persisted and encouraged them to try other different foods like spaghetti and pizza. Slowly and over time, I managed to get them to adjust to new tastes and flavours.

Clothes were washed by hand in those days as there were no washing machines. Mum used an old-fashioned clothes washer which was a wooden-framed contraption with a thick strong weaving glass within. The clothes were rinsed with soap suds and rubbed back and forth. This scrubbing and rubbing process was hard and laborious work when just using your hands. She usually used warm soapy water to rinse and then soak the soiled clothing. She would then wash the clothes according to how dirty they were cleanest first with the grubbiest last. The soaking-wet clothing would then be formed into a roll and twisted by hand to wring out the water. The wringing machine would then be used to rinse out the excess water. To help reduce the labour on the hands, the wringer/mangle used two rollers under spring tension to squeeze out the water. Each piece of clothing would be fed through the wringer separately and I often helped Mum to fold the wet clothes ready for 'wringing', after which we would hang them up on the washing line to dry. The first wringers were hand-operated, but they eventually became a powered attachment which was affixed above the washer tub. When Mum eventually got a small spin dryer, it sometimes danced around the kitchen!

Some friends of mine said they had always admired my mother because of her lovely personality and said she deserved to have the best in life after looking after my family. She always provided food and snacks for my friends and made sure all our visitors were comfortable. She was the most perfect, generous, loving person, the type who would buy us little presents for birthdays and Christmas. She would buy us comics too like the *Beano*, *Dandy* and *Beezer*. I used to love reading of Desperate Dan and Dennis the Menace and Gnasher his dog. Yet although we were hard up, we always had love. One of the things I distinctly admired about Mum was that she never spoke badly about any member of the family. She would tell us off though, if any one of us used a swear word; she loathed swearing in the house. No swearing was one of her ground rules and woe betide anyone who crossed Mum on this. But in all, she was never anything but a very dutiful mother. Bless her; we all adored her.

Christmas was a special time for us and every year we would have a family gathering, exchanging presents and eating traditional seasonal foods. Turkey, roast beef and vegetables were always on the table. Every December, Dad used to bring home a pine tree which Mum loved to decorate with tinsel that had been kept especially for the occasion. Mum would also set up a small nativity display of the birth of Jesus, along with animals, next to the tree so that there was a true feeling of Christmas spirit. In the evenings, the hall lights were switched off and the Christmas tree lights were lit up. My parents would have a drink, unwind and listen to their favourite old records, sometimes singing along.

My family would visit Auntie Glad and Uncle Taffy in Edmonton every fortnight on a Sunday and they would visit us too. When they came to us, Philip, Paul and I would go up to Uncle Taffy asking him for pocket money and he would give us half a crown each. Uncle Taffy would ask us questions to find out if we'd been good or if we had stories to tell about school. When we went to Edmonton, I remember we used to run round the garden playing all sorts of games whilst the adults engaged in hours of discussion, often reminiscing about the good old times. Auntie Connie, Uncle Walter and Auntie Maud would also join in the family gathering even though they had no children of their own.

At home, when she needed space and time to herself, Mum would play the Steinway piano in the private lounge and enjoy the occasional vodka and lemonade. She used to sing a lot when we were young and I realised that playing the piano was a kind of therapy for her. When she was upset, or when she was having a bad day, she would play the piano alone. She taught me how to play a tune or two and I can still remember playing them. She really adored the Steinway and for me, being Deaf, it was a very powerful instrument; I could feel the strong vibrations that ran through it when it was played. The keys were made of ivory and the body was strong sturdy rosewood. Mum looked after the piano lovingly and would give it a good polish with furniture wax. When we fell on hard times and had to sell the piano, Mum was heartbroken - she never recovered from the loss of her prized piano.

Ballroom dancing was another of Mum's keen interests. She and Dad used to go to the Tottenham Empire in North London to dance with their friends and at times like Christmas or a family party, there would always be dancing. Mum loved dances such as the waltz, the foxtrot, the Gay Gordons and whatever else was fashionable at the time. She and Dad would go ballroom dancing whenever they could. They always enjoyed being with other people and Mum would put on a little make up, rouge and lipstick to look good. With her fashionable taste in clothes she would appear most attractive.

In 1960, *Coronation Street* became Mum's favourite TV drama. She loved to watch all the characters and avidly followed the fortunes of Ena Sharples, Elsie Tanner and Annie Walker. Her favourite film was the American Civil War epic *Gone with the Wind* starring Clark Gable and Vivien Leigh; a classic from 1939 which told of a doomed romance during the American Civil War. Mum loved that film so much she saw it at the cinema 10 times!

Another favourite pastime Mum had was crosswords and she would regularly enter crossword competitions; she would phone her sister Connie frequently to compare crossword answers. Every day, Mum and I would complete the crossword from the *Daily Mirror* newspaper and even on a Sunday we would do the *News of The World* crossword together. She never won any of the competitions, but I managed to win one in the *Sunday Mail!* We loved to sit doing crosswords as it was quality time for both of us. I still do them today, though I find some quite challenging!

I know Mum had a good life and that she enjoyed being with the family; she was always there for us and we will always remember her as a good mum. My Uncle Don said to me a couple of years ago that I was the spitting image of my mother and that I reminded him of days gone by.

Mum suffered from senile dementia in later years and had to be moved to a nursing home. Nevertheless she was happy there and was loved by the staff: singing, sharing jokes and playing dominoes. Every time I visited, she would proudly show off her awards for dominoes, which was surprising as she had never played dominoes before! Family members were sad when she began not to recognise them in the later stages of her illness. We would bring in photographs to try and jog her memory and reminisce over events long gone. But she wasn't well - when she was diagnosed with dementia it was found that she also had type two diabetes, high blood pressure and bronchitis.

Sadly, Mum died peacefully in her sleep in November 2008.

3

My Family

Through research, I found out that my mother had changed her name by deed poll from Griffiths to Kenneth. It was confirmed in the Registry on 2nd July 1945. I believe that this was around the time my mother was five months pregnant with her first child, Ian. I think the reason she changed her surname was that at that time, unmarried pregnant women were labelled as 'shameful'. Having sex before marriage in those days just wasn't done and it was shameful for parents to have a daughter who was pregnant from a relationship with a married man. As it was, Mum was unable to marry Dad because he was already married. I have since been told that Dad had to endure a family dispute with his sisters - with their strong beliefs and family values, they disapproved of a single woman getting pregnant.

With the prevailing attitudes of the 1940s, Mum could have been sent to the workhouse, but Dad supported her all the way through and luckily she escaped such a fate.

My brother, Ian, was born in November 1945 in Derbyshire, where Mum had been evacuated to in order to escape the London Blitz. That was the year when the Second World War had come to an end. Half of all London schoolchildren and pregnant women were evacuated to the countryside, so they could be safe from air raids and bombings. They were billeted with families who were required to accommodate the newcomers.

Mum said she and other family members listened to the radio to hear the Prime Minister, Winston Churchill, speaking on the progress of the war. When the war eventually ended, Mum returned to London to lead a normal life though times were hard. The Government made it compulsory for everyone to be on what was called the 'national register'. The register held information for issuing identity cards, food, clothing and ration books. The Government also made proposals regarding how hospital services should be provided and from this, in 1948, emerged the National Health Service. Most families were struggling to get food for children and everybody had to use a ration book to obtain what limited food and drink was available. Butter, milk, cheese and sweets were in short supply, as were fruits such as bananas.

Three years after the war ended, my second brother Alan was born in October 1948. My third brother, Richard, was born in May 1952 and then came along my fourth brother, Philip, in September 1954. Finally, I was born along with my twin brother Paul in July 1956. We were all born at Hackney Hospital, East London, except Ian who was born in Derbyshire. Philip was diagnosed as deaf when he was 15 months old by our local GP, Dr McLaughlin. When Paul and I were born, Mum believed that we were also deaf and informed Dr McLaughlin accordingly. He assured Mum that we were not, but she was adamant because she said she could tell the difference between my hearing brothers and Philip, Paul and me. Mum was right when she confronted Dr McLaughlin again as the result of a hearing test came back as positive for deafness.

At that time we were living in the privately-rented ground floor flat in Eade Road, Haringey. We also had another family living with us temporarily. It was Mum's sister Gladys, with her husband Alfred and four children. We called Alfred 'Uncle Taffy' because he was a Welshman. Eade Road was a two-bedroom flat; there was no bathroom available, only a toilet which was located outside and at the back of the house. We had two huge reception rooms. The kitchen was very small and we used to have our baths by the coal stove where it was warmer. Every week, Paul and I would share the bath, filling the portable metal tub with boiled water heated on the kitchen stove. It sounds as if two families living in only a two-bedroom flat would be overcrowded, but we all managed very well I was told. Auntie Gladys' family lived with us due to the acute housing shortages caused by the war. They were re-housed under the Government's 'Homes for Heroes' scheme because Uncle Alfred had seen active service as a soldier. The Government and the Armed Forces saw to it that veterans and ex-soldiers were rewarded for their endeavours with new homes. Auntie Gladys, Uncle Alfred and their two children, Carol and David, eventually moved to their home in Edmonton where they lived for years. Their other two children, Valerie and Geoffrey, were born in Edmonton. Today, it amazes me that we were all crammed into that two-bedroom flat. In the upstairs flat was a couple called Margaret and Fred Piper, who had two British boxer dogs. They had no children of their own but were devoted to their dogs. I recall that not only was I terrified of the two boxers but my brothers were as well. They were vicious and tough-looking but really they made excellent guard dogs for us all. I remember they were a lovely tan colour with a bit of a whitish patch on their face. Every time any one of us made an entrance through the front door the dogs would be at the top of the stairs barking and watching our movements. We would go upstairs to greet them where they would lick our hands and faces.

Fred Piper used to breed chickens in the back garden. He often asked my brothers Ian and Alan to help him round up his wayward birds when they were loose from the coop. Ian and Alan used cardboard boxes with a flap and strings attached as a makeshift trap so that when a chicken went inside for food, the string was pulled and the flap closed, trapping the bird. Sometimes Ian and Alan would make clucking noises and the chickens would enter the box without any hesitation! Then they would be put back into the coop and Fred would be happy with their work. Fred and Margaret would often provide us with fresh eggs from the chickens.

Whilst we were living in Eade Road, we had lots of pets including a dog, cat, hamster, goldfish, tortoise and a budgerigar and of course the two boxer dogs that lived upstairs. Mum hated it when our pet budgie Joey was let out of the cage in the living room, because she didn't like to see its wings flapping around. She would put a towel over her head and hold it fast until Joey was safely back in the cage. My brothers teased Mum, encouraging Joey to land on her head but she wouldn't have any of it. Dad used to coax Joey onto his shoulders, kissing his beak and talking to him. He would pretend to have a serious conversation with Joey, and used to say the budgie would accuse my brothers of behaving badly and being naughty!

We had a huge garden and a small stream at the back that ran down to the River Lea. There was a massive apple tree on the right side of the garden and my brothers made a tree house there. They would spend hours climbing up into their makeshift eyrie, looking out at the views and playing games. Every year we would collect apples from the tree to make delicious apple pies for our family and the Pipers.

In the harsh winter of 1963, there was snow everywhere. The snow was about three feet deep and the ice was thick enough in places for people to skate on. I could see icicles hanging from many of the roof gutters. Some of these were as much as three feet long!

Ian and Alan wanted a sledge but we didn't have one. So they used Mum's best metal tea tray as a sledge in Finsbury Park. There was much fun to be had bolting down the slopes on the tray sledge and there were dozens of other children doing the same. The tray had pictures of beautiful swans on it, but by the time it was quietly returned to the kitchen it was battered beyond recognition! Ian and Alan got a well-deserved slap on the back of their heads for the damage caused. Undeterred, my brothers and I would make snowmen outside the house and we even made a huge snowball that we rolled down the hillside.

When my twin brother Paul was three years of age, he was involved in a horrific road accident. At about this time, Philip, Paul and I often played hide and seek and we hid in various places inside the flat. We would soon run out of hideouts and would venture outside. On one occasion, it was Paul's turn to look for Philip when, in his excitement, Philip ran across the road without thinking. Paul instinctively followed him and I did the same. I didn't see what happened, it was all a blur, but I remember a motorbike suddenly screeching past, down on its side with smoke coming out of the exhaust pipe. Paul was hit and thrown some 20 feet through the air. The motorcyclist got up, picked Paul up and cradled him as he hurried to our house where he put him on the floor in the hallway. He was trying to resuscitate him whilst Philip and I watched in dumbfounded horror. I remember clearly the right side of Paul's forehead where a lump of skin was hanging off, revealing a gleam of white bone underneath. Blood was everywhere. My eldest brother Ian arrived on the scene and shoved me and Philip into the living room, shutting the door to prevent us from becoming further traumatised.

Alan and Richard were in the garden when they heard commotion and people shouting from the front of the house.

They rushed to see what was happening and were shaken to find their brother covered in blood and his body looking limp. Paul was rushed to the Prince of Wales Hospital in Tottenham where he received emergency treatment. He had two broken legs, a broken arm and he was in a coma for a short while. I remember at visiting times in the hospital, Philip and I used to ride a child's tricycle around the ward, whilst Paul lay in bed with his legs hoisted up to a winch like some awkward Egyptian mummy. His arm was up in a winch too! If it wasn't all so awful it would have been comical. Paul stayed in hospital for six months until he was fully recovered. To this day, he still bears a scar on his forehead from the handlebar of the motorbike. The motorcyclist was naturally very upset at the scene and my parents were very supportive of him. I remember he came to visit us at times to see how we all were.

In the same year that Paul's accident happened, I recall that I had a lot of pain in my left ear and had to be admitted to hospital. Mum was with me when we went into the hospital lift which was very old and had heavy metal bars securing the doors shut. Later, I talked to Mum about this and she said that I was only three years old and that I had to have a minor operation to remove mastoids from behind my ear. She asked me how I remembered all this and I told her that it was because I was scared of the metal bars in the lift!

Dad changed his job during the 1950s and worked at Hicks Machinery as an engineer, restoring heavy machine tools in a tiny workshop off Green Lanes. He also worked at nights and weekends as a barman in the Mildmay Tavern in Islington, and at The Albion on Albion Road, Stoke Newington. He used to earn this extra bit of money to provide for the family. When he came home from work, he would get annoyed with either Alan or Richard because they always had pop music blaring from Radio Luxembourg. Dad preferred to listen to other music when he got in and so he always had to re-tune the radio.

Richard loved to listen to pop music every day. He would use a knife and fork to drum on a table. Occasionally, I would go into the kitchen where Richard was listening to the radio and I would ask him what was on the radio. He would say it was 'just music'. But eventually Richard became curious about my deafness and started to test me. He would say, 'There's the doorbell, go and see if someone is at the door.' I would dutifully go out to answer the door but, of course, there was no one there. I would get up again, but still there would be no one there. I would return to the kitchen and Richard would just laugh at me because he was teasing my deafness. This really wound me up. Eventually I figured out when there actually was someone at the door and then I would open it. Richard asked me how I knew the doorbell had sounded. I refused to tell him so that he wouldn't have the satisfaction of knowing, but he was always curious to see how I knew the door bell was ringing. One day I relented and told him; I would watch our cat Blackie because whenever the doorbell sounded, she would look directly at the front door and twitch her ears!

As our family had grown, my parents applied to the council for a bigger house. Consequently we moved from Haringey to Stoke Newington in 1961, where we were provided with a five-bedroom house in Bethune Road. There was a real wow factor to this house for us because it had three floors, stairs and a huge attic. On the first-floor landing, there was a spare living room where we would entertain. Mum's piano was there and Dad's bar was in the corner. The lounge also had access to an outside balcony from which we could see along Bethune Road.

Our next-door neighbour was a lady named Rita. Mum got on especially well with her and they would natter away for hours, reflecting on all the local 'goings-on' and dissecting the latest gossip. They remained friends for over 40 years.

During the 1950s and 1960s, there was a sizeable Orthodox Jewish community in Stoke Newington. The men wore long black robes and fur hats and the ladies wore wigs. Many of the married men shaved their heads as was the Jewish tradition. Although we were culturally different, we felt that we were similar to them in that we too were a very tight-knit family. The Jews originated from Russia and were refugees who had emigrated to England at the time of the First World War.

We had a Jewish family living opposite to us at number 35. They had a huge cherry tree in their garden which was close to the garden wall. The father wasn't happy with the local kids invading their garden to pick his cherries. I remember once, Ian chased off two young men who were trying to climb over the wall to 'scrump' the cherries. Suffice to say, we were very pleased with the bags of succulent red fruit we were given every year!

We would frequently go down to Clissold Park to play and walk Polly, our dog. One day, my brothers and I were told off because Polly jumped into the pond for a swim and the park attendant wasn't very pleased. The attendant said it disturbed the ducks, swans and other wildlife but we always knew Polly would never harm them. Polly would make a habit of jumping into the pond whenever we went to the park and we would run off when we spotted a marauding park attendant! Eventually, Polly would catch up with us, stinking of pond water and needing a bath.

Clissold Park had many different types of trees, a cafe and a mini animal zoo. By the entrance to the park from Grazebrook Road, there stood a massive oak tree, its branches veering out in different directions. It was a beautiful tree and it rose up high into the sky looking really grand. I used to sit by this tree for hours with Polly just watching the world go by. I must have been 11 or 12 at the time, my mind immersed in a private world of grass, dirt and creepy crawlies. I would examine each blade of grass, studying the tiny dew drops. The dirt was incredibly warm and the grass seemed to sway softly in the breeze as I whiled away the time with Polly sitting beside me.

It was the most relaxing time I ever had and it would only be later that I would realise that I'd been there an hour or so. Sometimes I would spot a sparrow or a blue tit hop from one branch to another. At other times, my brothers and I would go to a different park, Finsbury Park, another park with lots of playground facilities for children which was very popular with families.

Just over a year and a half ago, I was cat-sitting for two weeks at a friend's flat just behind Stoke Newington Church Street. I was amazed to see how different the area had become with its eclectic range of pubs, restaurants, trendy clothes shops and more. Stoke Newington Church Street has got a real 'village-y' feel about it, which is nice if you want to escape from hectic London life. I still love everything about this area which has easy access to the city or the West End by the number 73 bus service. Alan used to be a driver on the number 73 bus which would take you all the way to Oxford Street and Bond Street. In Stoke Newington High Street now, there's a strong Turkish feel. There are lots of kebab shops, cafes, banks and grocery stores which are all owned by Turks and thrive in the area.

When I was a teenager, Philip, Paul and I used to call at the neighbours' to ask for Saturday day jobs like gardening or cleaning cars for pocket money. One day, we were in the Rosenfelds' house a few yards away in Grangecourt Road and they asked us to do some gardening, like cutting the grass with shears. I noticed a couple of wigs on the clothes line and wondered why there were there.

Puzzled by this, I approached Mum and asked what it was all about. She explained to me that it is a Jewish tradition for the married women to shave their heads and wear wigs. Mum regularly hand washed these wigs for Mrs Rosenfeld and hung them up on the washing line to dry. I was shocked at the time, but soon became adept at peering under passing hairdos and checking 'wig or not?'!

In the early years, I remember my parents had a huge Silver Cross pram. It was a strong black metal pram with chrome trimmings, spoked wheels and solid rubber tyres. All my brothers and I were carried in that pram when we were babies. When the pram was no longer needed, my brothers made a trolley kart out of wooden planks and used the pram wheels, along with an old skipping rope for steering. It was a fantastic kart and we rode it all around the local streets. We all took turns pushing and driving the kart, often having mishaps and crashing up against walls as we had no brakes. Sometimes we raced against the other local families who also had such karts, even having competitions. Like most other children in the 50s and 60s, we were always playing in the street - football, cricket, hopscotch and glass marbles.

There was a fantastic playground near to us in Downhill's Park, Tottenham, called the 'Model Traffic Area'. It was the only one of its kind in England and we loved it! It featured radio-controlled road safety systems and we would ride around it on hired bicycles. The mini traffic lights would be in use and there would be lots of other road signs displayed. It was designed to help develop road safety skills and we would regularly go there on Sundays to ride our bicycles and meet other children. Alan, Philip, Paul and I really enjoyed going there. The routes were quite straightforward and so I felt quite safe. The Model Traffic Area was a very popular facility for the children in Tottenham in the 1960s and for us, it was just a quick bus ride down from Stoke Newington.

Road safety became an issue for me one day when I went to get an ice cream. I remember Mum saying, 'Ding dong ding dong! It's the ice cream van!' and she gave me money to get myself a cone. I was across the road in a flash, got my ice cream and hurtled back the way I'd come. Suddenly a police car screeched to a halt inches in front of me! I dropped the ice cream in shock. The policeman driving the car got out and started to question me, but in my state of shock I couldn't understand him. He realised I was Deaf and asked me if I could lipread him if he spoke slowly. I just nodded, not saying a word. He asked me where I lived and I pointed meekly over the road. He took me to Mum and I could see they were discussing my road awareness given how vulnerable I was. I was lucky not to get told off, but was reminded that because of my Deafness, I needed to be extra careful. It was a day I will never forget and the image of a big police car stayed with me for a long time.

We were always a close-knit family. Every year we went on our holidays in a hired Volkswagen camper. We went to places like Butlins holiday camps or camping sites. The camper had an extension on the roof and was big enough to fit our family of six. If a Volkswagen wasn't available then sometimes we would hire a Bedford van. There were lots of seaside resorts and places we visited during the Easter and summer holidays. We went everywhere and when we went up to Scotland, we would stay with Dad's relatives.

We had one holiday in Scotland where we'd pitched our huge family tent on the sand dunes near the sea at Monifieth. We'd all visited Dad's sister Auntie Agnes at her place for the day and had enjoyed a hearty tea with her family. Upon returning to the tent, we unzipped the front cover to find that there were hundreds and hundreds of spiders crawling inside. We were terrified and there was no way we were going to sleep there for the night. Auntie Agnes was very surprised to see us all on the doorstep again!

I remember a story about staying near a farm somewhere in Devon when a bull was very near the campsite. Paul and I were taking a walk in the countryside and we must have crossed the wrong path towards the farm and the bull noticed us walking. The bull became aggravated, possibly due to us intruding on his territory, but we were blissfully unaware of what was going on. As we continued walking along we could not hear the bull's snorting and the beginnings of a rampage. My other brothers Ian, Alan, Richard and Philip could see from the other end what was going on; they were horrified to see the bull and were trying to warn us by waving their hands by the gate, but then had to wave their coats at us to get out of the field. I thought it was nice of them to wave to us but could tell by their faces they were anxious. Paul and I looked behind and suddenly the bull was heading for us. Luckily we ran for our lives and jumped over the massive gate and landed on our backs in the mud! Our clothes absolutely stank! Even though Mum was annoyed at what happened, she eventually managed a laugh. She was the one who had to bravely hand wash our clothes when we got back to the campsite.

I was told one day that in the remotest hills of the Highlands of Scotland, my brothers Alan, Richard, Paul and I were walking along when suddenly Alan and Richard heard the flapping of wings and noticed a huge golden eagle flying towards us. They ran and pushed me and Paul flat down on the grass because the eagle was making a swoop on one of us, baring its razor-sharp talons. We were saved but I really never remembered that story. I still don't know whether Alan or Richard are telling the truth when they talk about it.

Every year we holidayed as a family either in Scotland or somewhere by the seaside in England or Wales. We would travel by camper van and stay in the tents. We always had fun and lots of different adventures: flying kites, rolling down the hills, playing games and running about in the remote countryside. In the fields, sometimes we got our arms and legs covered in painful lumps running through ivy or nettles. Mum would put calamine lotion on our arms and legs to ease the nettle rashes. Paul and I were always the most adventurous as we liked to explore things, but Philip always remained close to Mum wherever she was.

Sometimes we stayed in a caravan at Butlins in Clacton-on-Sea. There was always something to do: amusements, slot car racing games, sports activities and entertainment at the club in the evenings. My parents loved to drink and dance while we sat by the table and watched. We made our own fun with other people we met and during the summer of 1966, we stayed up late to watch the World Cup final between England and Germany. The place erupted in excitement when England won and beat the Germans 4-2. There were raucous celebrations long into the night and the atmosphere was of one great big party!

On one occasion we took our Wolseley to Wales. We were towing a trailer and as we went along the M5, a police car stopped us. The officers fined us for overtaking in the outside lane which was forbidden with a trailer. Dad was muttering under his breath and I knew he was swearing because he didn't want to spend his hard-earned wages on a traffic fine! When we arrived at the camp site in Aberystwyth, we excitedly put up the huge canvas tent.

A few hours later, Paul and I were playing up on a hill when I got hit by a camper. The wheel accidentally ran over my foot and caused both massive swelling and heavy bruising. My foot had a huge black patch and I had to hobble down towards the tent and alert Dad. In a mad rush, Dad bundled me into the car and then drove off immediately to the hospital. But alas, he had forgotten to unleash the washing line which was attached to the tent. Suddenly the tent came down in a crash of canvas and bent poles, our washing dumped on the ground. Without hesitation, Dad released the washing line from the roof rack and drove off. Mum was suitably unimpressed as she sat in her deckchair and watched the chaos unfold. I had my foot checked and it was confirmed that it was bruised but luckily no bones were broken. Every four hours I had to take paracetamol to ease the pain. After the hospital visit and fearful of the next disaster, Dad decided to go home. The tent was a write-off and was impossible to repair so we had to throw it away!

That holiday in Wales was to be the last family gathering because Ian, Alan and Richard began to lead separate lives with their partners. Paul and I continued to holiday together, often going abroad with friends. My parents accepted that we were grown up now and that we all wanted to do our own thing.

For years, my parents always went on holiday in Great Britain but eventually they had a chance of a lifetime to go on holiday to New Zealand in 1978 over the Christmas period. My parents were worried about me being left alone with Philip, but I said I would be fine. However, to reassure them, I went to stay with Alan and checked on the house from time to time

Mum and Dad had a fabulous time - they stayed with Ian and his family for three months and they loved it all. They especially enjoyed being taken around the North Island by Ian, Lillian and the children. When they came back, they looked tanned, fit and in the prime of their lives!

4

Deaf Identity

As I explained earlier, Ian, Alan and Richard were all born hearing whereas Philip, Paul and I were born deaf. It seems that there was a history of deafness in the family and we had genetically inherited the condition.

Ian, Alan and Richard accepted our Deafness without question but always used the oral method when communicating with us and within the family. They never quite accepted that British Sign Language (BSL) was part of our life and that it was our preferred means of communication once we had left secondary school. Time after time I would badger them that signing was vital to us, but they just used to shrug their shoulders and say, 'You lip read so well!' Looking back, I think they were too embarrassed to sign, especially in public.

Many years later, Mum told me that both she and Dad had been encouraged by the local education authority not to use BSL as it was deemed 'not appropriate' and that the oral method was the best way for deaf children to communicate. In the 1960s and 70s, oralism was the communication method prescribed in most deaf schools. I guess this is why my hearing brothers got the impression that using sign language wasn't the right thing to do.

At the natural heart of every Deaf community is its sign language. This expressive and visual language embodies the thoughts and experiences of its users and is rich in Deaf culture and heritage; there is something we all share together through our language. All Deaf people have their own signing skills and styles, reflecting the different backgrounds and areas from which they have come. Deaf people learn their sign language style from others and copy different signs, handshapes and movements. In this way, Deaf people develop skills, fluency and articulation in British Sign Language or Sign Supported English.

I believe that Deaf people who use BSL are more positive, confident and well-rounded than those who don't sign. Native signers are invariably Deaf children of Deaf parents or Deaf children who learned to sign when they were very young at Deaf schools where there was a positive attitude towards BSL. It seems to me that the attitude of some Deaf people who have good English skills and who became Deaf after the age of five tends to be one that rejects the use of BSL in schools, seeing it as stupid and unnecessary. I believe that this has, in turn, influenced the thinking of some hearing people who see BSL as daft and its users as 'Deaf and dumb'.

Yet BSL is a language in its own right with an extensive and rich vocabulary. And whilst in the past this language was thought by some hearing social workers, educationalists and church ministers of the Deaf to be improper, it has evolved over time to be become the preferred language of choice for many profoundly Deaf people, a language of which they are hugely proud and staunchly defend.

Some Deaf BSL users acquire their BSL skills after joining their local Deaf club. These people tend not to be fluent as they have learnt later in life and have missed the vital formative years so important in learning any language. Yet they will admit that BSL is the natural language of the UK's Deaf community and that its use is a powerful glue that results in the free flow of unrestricted and relaxed exchanges of ideas, thoughts and feelings amongst the members of the Deaf community.

Many Deaf signers still assume that BSL is to be used only at home or in Deaf clubs whilst an alternative style of signing, such as Sign Supported English, is preferable to BSL in public places. Naturally, today, it is bewildering for some Deaf BSL users to be told that BSL is now a 'real' language and that since March 2003 it has been officially recognised by the UK Government as a language. The campaign for recognition took many years and culminated in a rally at Trafalgar Square that saw 3,000 Deaf people march to Downing Street to hand over a petition to the former Prime Minister, Tony Blair. I was there - it was an incredible feeling marching, signing together, being part of an amazing victory that saw BSL recognised at long last.

From a very early age, I wore hearing aids. I first had them when I started at the London Fields Primary School. I was encouraged to wear hearing aids to help me hear environmental noise around me and to help improve my speech. Mum worked ceaselessly to teach us to speak properly and also made sure we pronounced words carefully when we had conversations at home.

Hearing aids are basically amplifiers and they are supposed to improve the auditory experience of the hearing-impaired child. The quality of this hearing experience gives the child an opportunity to 'hear' things and therefore helps them develop spoken language. A child's language development proceeds more rapidly in the early years of life and whilst a hearing aid does not restore a child's hearing to normal, it does provide an experience of sound that would be otherwise unheard. There is no doubt that hearing aids play a vital role in the child's sensory stimulation and contribute enormously to subsequent linguistic development.

I wore hearing aids from the age of five up until about thirty when I stopped using them; I found my inner ears became dry and sore from the plastic ear moulds that fit into the ears. I also suffer terribly with tinnitus - the sensation of noises within the head and ears. This has really tormented me and I've tried all sorts of treatments but there is no known cure; one can only learn how to cope with the noises. At one point I was told that tinnitus can be triggered by stress and that it's important to relax. Many people manage their tinnitus by listening to the radio or to music which in effect masks the intrusive noises. I can use headphones but have to be at home with my powerful hi-fi to get any sense of relief. I guess it's better than nothing and certainly better than the suggestions I got at the Ear, Nose and Throat (ENT) Department at St George's Hospital. After assessing my tinnitus, they gave me a video which showed water dripping into a lake and making ripples. There was also a bird flying round and whilst it was all pleasant to watch, regrettably it didn't do anything for my tinnitus!

I can remember when I was very young, about four or five years of age, Paul and I would be taken to the ENT hospital on Gray's Inn Road, King's Cross, for our six-monthly check-up and hearing test. At the reception area, there was a children's play area with a huge rocking horse. Philip, Paul and I would always spend our waiting time rocking and playing on this horse.

Mr Walker was a consultant professor and an expert audiologist. He would assess deaf children and give them regular hearing tests, recording the results on an audiogram, a graphic record of the test. The actual hearing test itself involved an audiologist using test equipment that made a range of high and low frequency sounds, through a set of headphones, which the patient acknowledged by flicking a switch.

Mr Walker used all sorts of different kinds of sounds such as a drum, whistle, bell, metal objects etc., all at different tones and pitches, to see if we could hear any of them. My audiogram told me that I could hear noises above 72 dB (decibels). Given that mild hearing loss is classified as being between 25-40 dB, moderate at 41-70 dB, severe at 71-95 dB and profound being anything greater than 96 dB, you can see that I was classified as severely deaf.

Mum had the right attitude towards Deafness and to us as Deaf children. For this I'll always be grateful as I've seen that some parents are just not aware of how to handle the challenge of a Deaf child. I have heard of and met many Deaf children who have been neglected or abused by parents or family members because either communication was non-existent, or the family didn't know how to handle them. They saw their child as 'handicapped' and felt unable to cope with them.

I know my Mum and Dad had regular contact with the National Deaf Children's Society (NDCS) and much appreciated the support they received from this organisation. Established in 1944, the NDCS is the only registered charity which specialises in caring for the needs of Deaf children and their families. It represents the interests of Deaf children in the UK and supports parents through a huge network of self-help groups. It provides a wealth of advice on all sorts of matters ranging from welfare and education through to health and audiology. The NDCS also gives grants for holidays, education and the purchase of specialised equipment for Deaf children and their families.

Aside from the NDCS, my parents received a lot of guidance from the local authority, general practitioners and health visitors. This gave them the opportunity to air any worries and to also work through the feelings of fear, guilt and confusion they had regarding Deafness in the family. The healthcare professionals at the ENT hospital were obviously trained to support the parents of Deaf children and their empathy is usually well received. I suspect my parents engaged in a lot of soul searching and questioned themselves about who was to 'blame' for the deafness in our family, but the matter was never discussed with us, and anyway, I can't see how they can be 'blamed' *per se*; genetics are genetics!

Teachers of the Deaf are specialists who are trained to teach and assist children to acquire spoken and written language. They have a unique set of skills and invariably have huge amounts of patience! This is because - and obviously so - Deaf children need a lot of specialised tuition with their speech, pronunciation and, of course, their general learning. There are most definitely differences between teachers of the Deaf and teachers of hearing children. The interaction between teachers of the Deaf and the children they teach is always going to be different from that of hearing teachers with their children.

Hearing children can listen with their ears and are usually quick to grasp what they are being taught whereas Deaf children often struggle. They rely on lipreading or use hearing aids and as a result, are slower to process information. Add to this that things often go wrong - lipreading is incredibly difficult and mistakes are commonplace. It is clear that teachers of the Deaf need to be persistent and measured; repetition is often the name of the game. As they grow and develop, Deaf children don't acquire the incidental information that surrounds them - adult conversation, the radio, TV and so on. The social programming of language for the Deaf children of hearing parents is miles apart from that of hearing children and so it is no surprise that teachers of the Deaf have a huge responsibility.

Looking back, I remember vividly the speech therapy sessions that Philip, Paul and I went through at London Fields Primary School. We had to wear awkward headphones and practise what the teacher wanted us to say. Using a piece of paper held close to our lips we had to pronounce the letter 'p' in such a way that the paper moved backwards. For the letter 'n' we placed two fingers on the nose, for 'k', two on the throat.

For 'l' we clucked our tongues in some strange elocution. It was all rather surreal.

From what I've seen and experienced, Deaf people have often been oppressed and marginalised by the hearing. I don't necessarily blame hearing people for this, but they frequently fail to grasp the intricacies of Deafness, Deaf culture and Deaf issues. My brothers hated hearing taunts like 'Deaf and dumb', 'Deaf mute', or 'Deaf as a post'. They protected me from this but of course, there were occasions when people would take the mickey out of Philip, Paul and I. Whilst family members were allowed to tease us about our Deafness because we were used to their remarks and knew that they understood our disability, derogatory comments from outsiders would be fiercely challenged by the rest of our family. Paul and Philip protected me but were able to take the mickey out of us themselves, sometimes calling us 'Oi!' rather than using our names. Acceptable to a point within our family but there were still times when this grated...

As a young person leaving school, I was certainly confused as to whether I belonged to the hearing or the Deaf world. I felt I was having an identity crisis, not knowing whether I should be hanging out with my hearing peers from school or my Deaf peers from the Deaf club. I wasn't sure how I felt about being Deaf and remember thinking, 'Am I different to hearing people?' In one respect I was certain I was Deaf because I realised there were many things that were different for me: I couldn't fully engage in conversations, I was left out of social gatherings, I couldn't follow films at the cinema and so on. For hospital, doctor or dental appointments I needed an interpreter. As to the number of times I got on the wrong train having missed tannoy announcements - well ... let's not get into that!

To address matters, Paul and I went to the St John of Beverley Deaf Club in Green Lanes, Haringey. Here we made new friends and shared our mutual feelings on identity, communication and belonging. Paul himself was struggling with his own identity and whilst we talked through the experiences that were affecting us - sometimes funny, sometimes sad - there was a welling anger between the two of us - anger and frustration directed at those whose ignorant attitudes disenfranchised us. To continuously challenge ignorance is draining; it never ends, but there were times when we were able to get the message across, to enlighten hearing people as to our language, culture and being.

Reflecting on my identity challenges, I am glad I made the decision to be 'Deaf'. It is where I am, what I understand and where I belong. A lot of the other pupils who went to the same school as me had the same identity crisis. Some chose not to immerse themselves in the Deaf world, preferring instead to be 'hearing'. It seems to me that these individuals actually had very mild hearing loss and so were better able to adjust to the audio demands of the hearing world, but for Paul and me, we were glad we could share our experiences, challenges and hopes with our Deaf peers.

And how times change; in the 1970s, Paul and I sometimes had great difficulty in contacting our Deaf friends as we did not have the advantages of computers, e-mails, Facebook and mobile phones. Frustratingly, we had to rely on hearing people to make telephone calls for us. The Friday night gathering or some other social activity always meant involving a hearing person. This was time-consuming and tedious in the extreme. Today, modern technology has gone a long way to improve Deaf people's access to wider society. It's great to be able to contact other people using video technologies or computers. Independence at last!

5

Education

Ian, Alan and Richard went to Woodberry Downs School which was about a mile away from our home in Stoke Newington. It would take them about 20 minutes to walk there. Philip, Paul and I went to Haverstock Comprehensive School near Camden Town where there was a Partially Hearing Unit (PHU). The red brick, three-storey building had been built in Victorian times and has since become Haverstock Business Enterprise College.

The journey took an hour and we had to travel by bus and Underground to get there. Haverstock had approximately 30 Deaf pupils in its PHU and, being the 'oralist' 60s and 70s, we were taught in spoken English and so had to learn to lipread. The use of British Sign Language was forbidden. Every one of us had to attend weekly speech therapy sessions which were, apparently, aimed at improving our speech and lipreading skills.

This aside, Haverstock School was quite an interesting place and, as it turns out, the learning seat of many famous faces such as the political brothers David and Ed Miliband, London Mayoral candidate Oona King and the singer Lily

Allen. If that wasn't enough, members of the north London rap band N-Dubz went there, as did the novelist Zoe Heller and a couple of premier league football players including John Barnes and Joe Cole. Quite a mix but sadly I never managed to bump into any of them!

There was recently an article in the *Mail on Sunday*, where one of Ed Miliband's classmates mentioned how Ed had been bullied at Haverstock because he was a 'very stuck up person looking down his nose at everybody'2. His brother, David, wrote an article which was also published in the *Mail on Sunday*, where he explained that in 1970, the parents of Haverstock pupils took it upon themselves to vote and decided that their children should not have to wear school uniforms. This was certainly progressive for the time and reflected the unique diversity and mix of both working and middle-class families.

Haverstock School wasn't easy for me - I was punished by the teacher when he caught me trying to use sign language to another pupil. He hit my hand with a ruler and it hurt! You just wouldn't get away with it today ... I was also teased and harassed remorselessly by one pupil who kept going on about my hearing aid. Jokes about the 'plug in my ear' abounded. I just wanted to die, but what made it worse was that when I confided my shame and humiliation to my good friend, she went off and hit one of my tormentors! I wasn't expecting that but I guess it taught him a lesson as he gave me a wide berth after that! Sadly, there's no getting away from the fact that there were a lot of vicious bullies around and the teachers were finding it difficult to handle matters. On the surface, things seemed to get settled quickly but beneath, things were simmering.

I only attended the PHU for my speech therapy sessions and for the rest of the time I was back in a classroom with hearing

---

[2] Taken from the *Mail on Sunday*, February 6th 2011, p.15.

children. What to say? I just got left behind. The teachers would just rattle on and forget I was there, making it impossible for me to lipread them. When they had so many other children to teach, it's no surprise the lowest denominator was dropped. My classmate Angela Chapman and I regularly sat together. She could see what was happening and so often handed me her written work so that I could copy it. The teachers cottoned on to this but were happy to let things be. But this didn't stop the agony. There were times when I felt too embarrassed to ask the teacher to repeat what they had just said and so if I got things wrong, the whole class would look at me. I would just stare down at the floor and implore it to swallow me. I later found out that the reason I was put in a hearing class was because, apparently, I was deemed to be 'intelligent' - whatever that means! Conversely, Philip and Paul spent the majority of their schooling in the Deaf unit.

Recent research has confirmed that most people (even those whose first language is English) can only understand 40% of what they lipread. Given this, it goes without saying that I felt I missed out at school. I had no support - no teaching assistant, nothing. Today, children who attend mainstream schools are supported by their own teaching assistants and are able to access communication support; whether it be British Sign Language or Sign Supported English. Their education and life prospects will be infinitely greater than those I had.

As for hearing aids, I don't think these helped much, as my terrible exam results show. I left school with just three CSEs in art, needlecraft and office practice. Yet these subjects helped me to acquire and learn useful practical skills. They are visual subjects and I was good at them because they were less theoretical than the likes of history, maths and English. These were all 'spoken' subjects and therefore difficult to follow, even with hearing aids. Though whether that made any difference remains to be seen - I wasn't even allowed to sit CSE examinations in history, mathematics, English and geography because I was told they were 'too difficult' for me.

My favourite subjects were art, office practice and sport. My art teacher, Mr Rolfe, was very supportive - he seemed to recognise some artistic talent and went out of his way to help me. His particular interest was pottery and so we worked together on a number of pottery projects - figurines and animals aplenty! I used special craft tools to produce my masterpieces and even entered local competitions, winning a prize or two. I felt comfortable with Mr Rolfe, who worked hard to get through to me, so when it came to the CSE art exam I pulled out all the stops. I made a real effort as I felt in his debt and that I owed him something for his endeavours. The result was that I achieved a CSE level 1 in art; thank you Mr Rolfe. As mentioned, I enjoyed sport and took part in cross-country runs every Tuesday. I was also captain of the rounders and the swimming teams. I took naturally to rounders and enjoyed the heavy 'thwack' of the bat hitting the ball. It was always hilarious to see the opponents falling over backwards as they stretched back to catch the ball!

It was only after I left school, aged 16, that my education proper really began. I went to Brixton College on a one-day-a-week English literacy and typewriting course. This ran for two years and was provided for by my employer, the Department of Education and Science. I had a sign language interpreter assigned to me for the course sessions and I found my English improved dramatically.

Leaving school was tough to begin with and I really missed my friends, but at the same time, it was exciting to be independent and earning a wage, even if it was just £10.00 a month. At last I was out in the big wide world and I was happy to help my mother with some rent money. She wouldn't let me pay her a lot but I was allowed to help with the shopping and bills. And for me, when I got the chance, I would hit London's

Oxford Street or King's Road, shopping for jewellery or clothes.

Nothing could beat that Saturday afternoon buzz!

At about this time, I was encouraged to join the local Deaf Club with some of my old school friends, and I finally ended up learning British Sign Language. It was easy for me to adopt the sweeping visuality of BSL with its use of whole body, face and hand movements. I found its use effortless.

Over time and from living with us, Ian, Alan and Richard developed their own approach to Deafness. They realised that they needed to employ distinct communication methodologies. They would try to gain our attention by waving or touching a shoulder. They would thump on the floor or throw little objects; rubbers, paperclips and crunched up paper frequently became airborne! Flicking the light switch was commonplace. They thought all of this was hilarious but of course, Deafness had made a huge impact on their lives too. Even my mother got into all this and used to thump the kitchen ceiling with a broomstick to wake me up in my bedroom above. Sometimes I would fall back asleep, but the thumping would continue until I was finally up. Nowadays I use a small vibrating alarm with the vibrator pad placed under the pillow. I'm pleased to say no more brooms!

One day I remember Richard was having a conversation with my mother about something or other. I watched but couldn't follow what they were saying. I asked them what they were talking about, and Richard said, 'Oh I'll tell you later'. This became a habit for him and sometimes he would forget to tell me; this would really wind me up and I would get quite annoyed. I made it clear to Richard that he would never understand how a Deaf person feels when they are told they'd be 'told later'! To get my own back I grabbed a set of headphones and forced him to wear them all day. I took advantage of this and started winding him up, pretending to talk to him orally, knowing that he wouldn't be able to follow me! I kept this up for quite some time and it really got to him, but I got what I wanted. He never ever left me out again and always sought to include me in family conversations.

Philip, Paul and I were equipped with Medresco OL56 body-worn hearing aids at primary school. The Medresco was the first transistorised aid provided by the National Health Service range until ear-level hearing aids became available in 1975. These were bulky and uncomfortable machines, such that we had to wear a breast strap and carry the hearing aid in a pocket. On one occasion when I was running for the school bus, the hearing aid fell out of the pocket and shattered on impact. I knew it was coming but when I got to school I was in trouble. Despite my protestations I got a real telling-off, the teacher lecturing me on how expensive the hearing aids were and how they should be looked after. Let's just say, I'd learnt my lesson and from then on I never wore the breast strap again, choosing to put on my hearing aid when I arrived at school.

The technology of hearing aids has clearly advanced and the digital aids of today are light years away from the ear trumpets and clunky wire boxes of old. Digital aids are now small devices that fit behind the ear and are powered by small batteries. If Deaf children are recommended for a hearing aid, they are sent for an audiology test to determine their actual level of hearing loss. Once this has been done, then the correct aid can be fitted. This will often involve attaching the aid to a special computer circuit so that the audiologists can ensure the aid matches the Deaf person's hearing capability; if the individual has difficulty hearing certain high frequencies, then the aid will amplify those frequencies and so on. There are other options for Deaf children today including cochlear implants - a surgical operation that implants a device to stimulate the auditory nerve.

For us, we wore hearing aids, and with the addition of

lipreading, we got by. Yet still within the family we faced challenges; Dad's Scottish accent made him difficult to follow at times and as mentioned before, Ian, Alan and Richard made little effort to learn British Sign Language. Again, not necessarily their fault as the oralist regime of the time positively dissuaded them from doing so. Even when I steeled myself to teach them a few basic signs, they shied away. An understanding of British Sign Language is absolutely essential for the communication and emotional well-being of Deaf children and exposure at a young age is vital. But in my experience this was sorely lacking in both the family home and the wider community.

6

Formative Years

I n my adolescent years, we always played with toys at home: spinning tops, yo-yos, board games, skipping ropes, Meccano, Lego - all of these and more. Philip loved using bows and arrows when we played Cowboys and Indians; he would turn the children's toys into feared weapons, removing the protective rubber from the tip of the arrow. Ouch - did they hurt!! Both Paul and I would end up with dozens of welts all over us! But it was all great fun and we spent many hours using old cardboard to build makeshift wigwams in the garden.

Out in the street, we would play cricket with our friends and neighbours for hours and hours. During the school holidays and at weekends we would bolt down our breakfasts and then shoot out to play all day till the streetlights came on. Tired, dirty and hungry, we would troop back to the house sporting the bruises sustained from the day's rough play!

This was the era when boys were boys and girls were girls! Lego, Action Man and soldiers were *de rigeur* toys for boys; dolls, dolls' houses and soft toys were essential for girls. I vividly remember one doll that was given to me for Christmas and which I absently put on the shelf in my room. I didn't really pay much attention to this doll until one day I saw a film on TV about scary dolls coming alive. I was terrified! I couldn't sleep at night and kept having scary nightmares! I couldn't get rid of the doll quick enough and so it was the Meccano and Lego I played with. These were, of course, all infinitely more interesting than dolls and so I spent many a happy hour with my brothers building and constructing all manner of things!

Richard's great love was bird watching and he would spend hours in Finsbury Park. Sometimes he would bring home birds' eggs for his collection. He would collect all sorts and use a needle to pierce the egg and drain the contents. He would then label the eggs - sparrow, starling etc. - and place them in a wooden box surrounded by wads of cotton wool. All of this is illegal today, rightly so, but at the time Richard was obsessive in his quest to grow his collection.

Whilst Richard was up to his egg-collecting antics, Philip, Paul and I would play ball or hog the park swings. I developed quite an interest in trees and used to explore all the different types in the park, my favourite being the oak trees, which were huge. They made excellent hiding places for hide and seek and we would shelter from the rain under them. In the autumn, we would enjoy the rustic colours and the cooler weather. There were also conkers - thousands upon thousands of them! We would collect them up to play conkers with other children. Philip and Paul would cheat by soaking their conkers in vinegar for a couple of hours which would make them moist and difficult to crack when playing. They would win loads of competitions against all the other children, becoming real conker champions!

The park was great fun for me and I would sometimes take our pet dog Polly there. A mongrel, she was very clever and would pull down the eiderdown in the morning, telling us she wanted walkies! She knew Philip, Paul and myself were Deaf and therefore very different from our other brothers because of our body language. She would paw us or run around for attention if she wanted something. She knew there was no point in barking and so only barked for attention with other members of the family!

I think Polly found me testing at times - there was one occasion when she was asleep and I noticed her whiskers. I gently pulled them and then trimmed them with a pair of scissors. When Mum called her she awoke and trotted into the kitchen in an unbalanced way. Let's just say I got mightily told off and I learnt that cats and dogs must have whiskers to help them balance. Fortunately they grew back shortly thereafter!

Another experiment I did with Polly was to dress her up! Once when out shopping I begged my mother for sunglasses. She bought them and I was so excited, because I had my very first pair of sunglasses. It felt great and I flaunted them in front of Paul trying to make him jealous as he didn't have any. Later, while we were playing with Polly, I wanted to see how the sunglasses would look on a dog. So I put them on her, balancing them on her soft nose. Paul put Mum's headscarf on her head and then she scampered off - she'd had enough!! Paul and I ran behind the dog trying to catch her, but it was too late - she had disappeared. About an hour later Polly returned to the house without the sunglasses and headscarf and I kept quiet about this without mother knowing. Paul looked at me in a rather quizzical way wondering where the sunglasses and headscarf were; I just shrugged and laughed.

I do remember one Christmas time when we were eating shelled nuts that had to be opened with a nutcracker. Dad accidentally dropped a walnut and Polly was straight in there, cracking the nut with her teeth, leaving the shell in bits around her! So that was it, every Christmas she would join us for nuts and more - including turkey leftovers with vegetables and gravy. And if that wasn't enough, mother would go to the butcher's every Saturday to buy a huge bone for Polly to bite and chew. It would last her a couple of days, with her chewing and grinding.

Her favourite place to sleep was on the sheepskin rug by the fireplace where we burnt coals and wood. Sometimes we had to drag Polly back from the fire as it would spit and crack, launching the occasional spark onto her rug. We didn't have central heating at that time and well, that fire could be really cosy.

Whilst all this 'dog-foolery' was going on, Alan and Richard were busy with the Boy Scouts. They were members of the local Scout group and spent much time acquiring a range of useful skills. From rope-work to cooking and first aid, the badges they wore with pride said it all! They were often away on camping weekends and they also got involved in fundraisers such as weekly jumble sales.

When Philip, Paul and I were very young, Dad was a regular at couple of local pubs - the Robinson Crusoe or the Albion. Every weekend on Saturday and Sunday lunchtimes we would wait in the car, bored, whilst he drank with his friends. For two tedious hours we sat there but when the Cokes and crisps appeared we would sit bolt upright and guzzle the fare! We enjoyed the secret snacks and this made all the waiting worthwhile. Meanwhile, back home, Mum would be cleaning the house and preparing a cooked dinner. Perhaps this was a ruse to get us all out of the house, perhaps there was method in the madness!

When domestic duties and chores required us to make ourselves scarce, Alan would use his pocket money to travel around London with his friends. Often on Saturday mornings they would go to Heathrow Airport to watch the planes taking off and landing. Sometimes they would go train-spotting, watching steam trains at station bridges or they would go to museums and other places of interest. Alan was very outgoing and he always loved to be travelling to and fro across London and beyond.

Occasionally, on weekends and as a family, we would venture down to Southend or Ramsgate for the day. On hot sunny days, Dad would hire deckchairs so that we could relax on the beach. I used to badger him for loose change so that I could enjoy the amusement arcades. We would all nudge the machines to get them to drop pennies onto to the shove level! Sometimes the machines would be alarmed and we would scarper off to another arcade before we got caught. In the evenings, we would have fish and chips for supper before heading home, sunburnt and tired.

On some occasions we would venture into the sea and I remember one time at Ramsgate when I went swimming. The weather was cloudy and warm when I entered the sea but suddenly it changed and I felt a current pick up. The waves started moving quickly and I began to panic. I was swallowing water and going under; frantically I kicked myself up to the surface and, through the waves, I could see Philip standing on the beach looking out at me. He waved frantically and at the same time, I forced myself to swim hard, managing to reach the beach. Philip was almost overcome with worry; he pulled me from the water, exhausted as I was, and embraced me. We decided not say anything as we didn't want to alarm our parents but it was a close-run thing. In due course and over time I totally forgot about the whole thing, but whenever I hear of drowning incidents featuring young people it all comes back.

Whenever we went to Margate, Mum would meet up with her best friend Dolly. Mum and Dolly had been close buddies before the war and they had kept in touch ever since. They would go out together for a couple of hours whilst Dad looked after us somewhere else. It was a welcome respite for Mum to spend some time away from the family and to be with an old friend for a change. She always came back to us light of foot and with a big bright smile! I can just imagine the two of them reliving their wartime experiences and gossiping about family and friends.

I can't remember exactly when it all started, but at some point during their teenage years, Ian decided to become a 'Rocker', Alan a 'Beatnik' and Richard a 'Mod'. Oh dear ... Ian and Richard would try not to end up fighting each other when they were with their respective Rocker and Mod friends! Ian had a motorbike and was the proud owner of a Triumph Tiger Cub 250cc. He was always working on this bike with his tools and equipment spilling across the driveway. Alan and Richard on the other hand shared a scooter, a Vespa G.S. 150cc. Philip, being younger, had to be satisfied with a Raleigh bike. For Paul and I there was no motorised transport and no bikes - we were far too young for all of that!

In the mid-1960s, our adolescent years, these conflicting British subcultures dominated. In later years, Richard explained to me what all this Rocker, Beatnik and Mod business was all about, that it was about identity, belonging, music and fashion.

These gangs of Mods and Rockers always seemed to be fighting. The newspapers and TV news bulletins were full of weekend or bank holiday riots in places such as Margate, Brighton and Bournemouth - Rocker gangs in their jeans and leather jackets giving the 'come-on' to the scooter-riding, sophisticated looking Mods with their sharp Burton suits and fishtail parkas; or the Mods giving the 'come-on' to the Rockers who rode heavy motorcycles and frequently scoffed at the Mods, who rode scooters. The Rockers considered Mods to be effeminate, snobbish charmers, whereas the Mods saw the Rockers as out of touch, rough and grubby. But as with all subcultures, they soon faded from view and the media turned its attention to the new fads - Hippies and Skinheads.

At about this time in the 1960s, Paul and I along with some other school friends would go shoplifting in Finsbury Park. We used to steal silly things like Ben Sherman shirts and Brut aftershave. After school, we'd get off at Finsbury Park and head into the shops. Well it was going to happen … one day I got caught. The shopkeeper or shop assistant - I don't know who it was - saw the crest on my school blazer and reported me to the head teacher. He immediately wrote a letter to my parents and, as expected, Dad went ballistic. He fixed me with his eyes and I knew it was coming. The pain from the leather belt as he walloped me was white hot in its intensity. Paul and I were sent to our rooms where we skulked in fear, hoping the punishment was over. The pain, embarrassment and contrition were total and complete. I've never shoplifted since.

Our next-door neighbours at number 39 were the Burns family: Mr & Mrs Burns, two sons - Bobby and Charles - and a daughter, Carol. Carol sometimes played with us whereas Bobby and Charles were Monopoly fanatics! They would often ask me to join them. Charles always, always won the game as he played regularly and was clever. He would quickly acquire Mayfair and Park Lane, putting on hotels so that he could extract huge sums of rent from us! Carol sometimes hung out with me and another friend named Susan who lived over the road in a flat. We just hung about as kids do but sometimes I felt I didn't fit in because they just didn't get Deafness.

Slowly but surely, Susan spent less and less time with us. We wondered why this was and then found out that she was having an affair with a married man who lived in a block of flats somewhere. It seemed the man wanted to end the relationship so Susan became depressed and withdrawn. She then shocked us all by committing suicide, jumping to her death from his top-floor flat. Susan's mother, who was single, was naturally heartbroken and we were all horrified - totally. Susan was only 16 at the time and was an only child. Her mother became a recluse and rarely went out, eventually moving away, never to be heard of again.

This was the first time I'd ever experienced anything like suicide and I wasn't quite sure what to do. I was stunned that something like that should happen to someone I knew and I never expected anything like that to happen in our area. Carol was very upset and angry with the man, saying that he'd got away with it all. I later heard that he had moved his family from the flat and moved on.

At the impressionable age I was, I found myself really spooked out by *The Exorcist*. This was back in the seventies when the film was all the rage. It attracted a lot of controversy and I could see why! After watching the film, I hardly had a good sleep for about two weeks.

You hear people talking about horror and ghost stories but you can never tell whether to truly believe what you've heard. But I still believe that it was a ghost that I saw one night...

I was reading a book in bed and was beginning to feel really sleepy. Just as I turned over to switch off the lamp I noticed a very young boy walking across the room. He looked sallow, emaciated and ill with a visible hunchback. The fear suddenly hit me and I froze, bug-eyed with terror. The hairs on the back of my neck stood up and my tinnitus screamed an incredible pulsing tone I'd not heard before. In a flash I pulled the blanket over my head and held it tight. I was sweating even though it was January and I kept my eyes shut. My head screaming and my heart pounding, I eventually let the blanket slip ... what was it I had seen?

In the same room but on another occasion, Paul's then-girlfriend was sleeping in my bed when I was away for the weekend. She reported seeing a young boy walking across the room. When I told Mum she didn't believe me. But later she relented and we went to Stoke Newington Town Hall to research the house's previous owners. It seems that the house was used as a private surgery which was run by two doctors. My bedroom was apparently a treatment room and it was there that a young boy had died. I was spooked, I freaked out when I learnt this, but I was told that if I put the Bible beside my bed it wouldn't happen again. I did that and sure enough, I never saw the boy again.

I didn't like being spooked and my brothers knew this. Once, I was just eight years and engrossed in a Hammer Horror vampire film that Dad had allowed me to watch when Ian came into the dark room and saw me cowering deep into the chair. As Christopher Lee attacked innocent people with his dark staring eyes, white-powdered face, red lips and huge fangs, Ian moved silently behind me. Knowing I couldn't hear him, he crept up and without warning bit my neck! I screamed, freaked, jumped up and hit the ceiling all in one! I ran off to my room and, well, it was years before I could watch a vampire film again!

Alan and Richard used to tease me and Paul mercilessly, trying to convince us that witches were real and that on Halloween night, they'd appear at midnight. One dark and wet Halloween night, Richard terrified the two of us, saying that a witch was coming to haunt us because we had been really naughty! I stayed awake all night in a frenzy of white fear awaiting the witch who, of course, never appeared.

Richard never gave up - witches, ghosts and more. He would taunt me and Paul remorselessly. Ian on the other hand used to boss me around, ordering me to clean and polish his boots with shoe polish. I reminded him of all this years later, but he denied it. I remembered it well because of the enduring smell of shoe polish! He went red in the face explaining himself in front of his wife Lillian and tried to make up some story about paying me pocket money! He never did, but then that's brothers for you!

7

Family Secrets

Finding out that Dad had been married before was a real shock. His first wife, Rosetta, died in 1964 at the age of 43 from a coronary occlusion - a partial or complete obstruction of blood flow in the coronary artery. Two years later and in secret, my parents married at the registry office in Stoke Newington Town Hall. The marriage certificate I found said that Mum's sister, Gladys, was the witness.

Hidden away in their bedroom drawer, the certificate had lain undisturbed and untouched, a testament to former lives. Once I'd overcome my shock I was in a dilemma as to what to do ... should I tell them what I'd found out or should I sit tight? In the end and some point later I blurted it out to my eldest brother Ian and his wife Lillian; they were incredulous. They didn't believe me at first but once it had all sunk in, they told me - in no uncertain terms - not to tell anyone and not to say anything. They didn't want to upset our parents and so we all decided to leave things as they were. My brothers and I will never know the truth. It was after all *their* secret and they did have a right to a private life.

Obviously - and even though they weren't legally married - Dad stood by Mum when she was pregnant with Ian. Looking back, Ian and Lillian believed it was my parents' wish not to reveal anything to us as a way to keep the family together. I accepted this and so kept the secret for years, knowing that my parents strongly and staunchly believed in the value of the family. I also understood that my parents wanted me and my brothers to believe that we were the perfect family unit. Sometimes when I think back, I am sure that Mum and Dad must have discussed all this in private.

What is odd is that before I knew all this, I would ask Mum where they got married and if I could have a look at the wedding photographs. There were photographs of my aunties' and uncles' weddings around the house but not my Mum and Dads'. I'm sure that at one point Mum said that the photographs had been destroyed in the war. Nevertheless, I would wonder and I think excitedly about silver or golden wedding anniversaries to come. But of course, there were no wedding photographs and seemingly no anniversaries. I later realised she had been avoiding the truth and that photos taken in 1966 would have revealed their ages.

Did our parents ever actually think about telling us the truth? Did one of them want to? Did they feel guilty or was there some sense of shame? Were they embarrassed that we were 'illegitimate' children - 'bastards'? I don't think there's any shame but now we'll never know. Though personally I just wish they could have been a little more open and honest.

Maybe it's my natural curiosity but I often wonder why Dad left his first wife and family behind. What was the real reason behind leaving? Did they fall out of love or was there a feud? It is possible that he did not love Rosetta or that there were family feuds in the past. I felt, and still feel, that we deserved to know the truth. Could it be our parents were waiting for us to bring the matter up in some casual conversation? Surely it wasn't really down to us?

I recall my parents going away for a couple of days - perhaps it was their honeymoon - and we all went to stay on a farm somewhere in Kent. I hated it there. The people who were looking after us barely knew us and were distinctly unfriendly. They told us not to touch anything, use anything. We couldn't move and were frozen like rabbits in headlights; not knowing what to do or where to go. I have a vivid memory of being upset and feeling neglected. When my parents came to collect us, I told Dad I hated it there. He reassured us that it wouldn't happen again.

Are families planned or do they just happen? I remember once asking my parents why they had such a large family. They said that it was because they wanted a daughter, so that was how I came about last with my twin brother. Did the fact that Dad had two daughters from his previous marriage influence his need to have one in his second family?

Dad's two daughters, Kay and Heather, had not been seen or heard of since he left his first wife, but there was a rumour from Dad's sisters in Scotland that Kay was living in London and Heather was living in America. Alan once mentioned that he and Ian were once with Dad at the Post Office and he was paying over maintenance money for the girls. Both Ian and Alan asked Dad what the money was for and to whom it was being sent, but he wouldn't tell them, telling them to 'be quiet!'

Did my brothers ever talk about all this between themselves or did they just ignore it? They must have been curious as to who this 'Kay' and 'Heather' were and why money was being sent to them. Did they ever question what Dad was doing and why he seemed to be hiding something from them? Did they ever think to ask Mum or did they realise she would be vague and evasive?

Today, I often wonder about Kay and Heather, our half-sisters. What do they look like? Do they resemble us? If we met them how would the meeting go? Would it be amiable? What if they didn't like us or we didn't like them? Or what if we all got on well and became close? What if I sensed an immediate connection with them - what would that mean? I've also wondered if they know about us. Would they want to meet us or would it be too painful for them because of what Dad did? Am I real in their lives, known about, talked about and cared for, or am I forgotten and hidden away like a terrible secret?

Sometimes I see a woman walking down the street or having a coffee in the cafe and I think, 'Is that her?' Or someone catches my eye; we fleetingly hold a gaze then break away. 'Is that my sister?' I think, 'Was she looking at me? Do we know each other?'

My brothers and I have occasionally discussed trying to find Kay and Heather but we decided against it as it would serve no purpose now. Or maybe we're just too scared to face reality? I guess we'll never know.

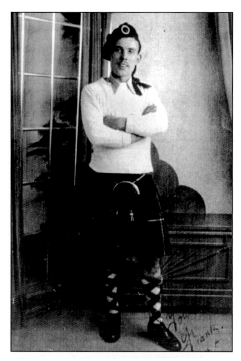

Dad at 19 years old in 1933 – Ever the proud Scotsman

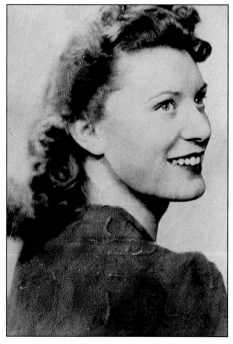

Mum at just 21 years old – 1941

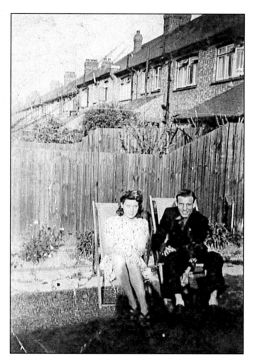

Mum & Dad pictured during the war years – 1942

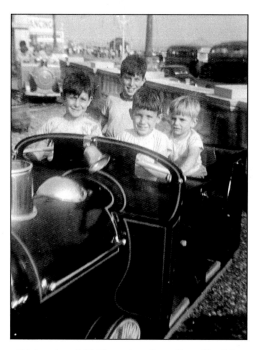

Alan, Ian, Richard and Philip enjoy the railroad! – Margate 1959

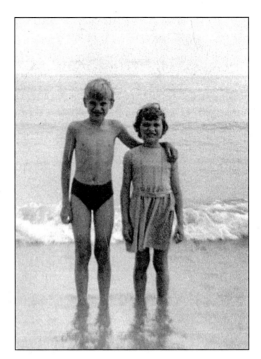

Philip and Sylvia take the waters! 1964

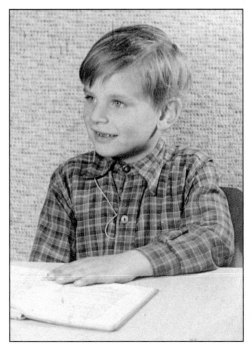

Philip aged 7 years at London Fields School – 1965

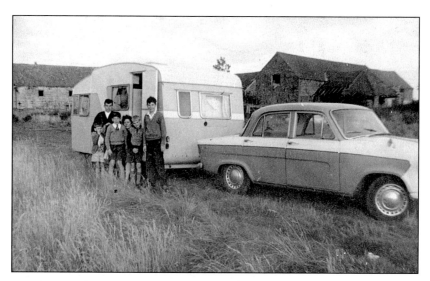

One of our exciting family holidays! Caravanning in Scotland

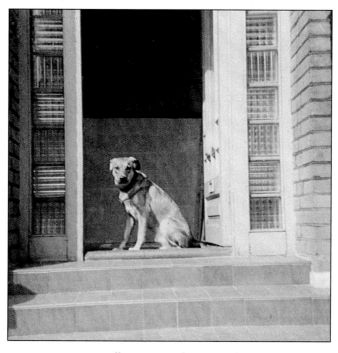

Polly at 37a Bethune Road

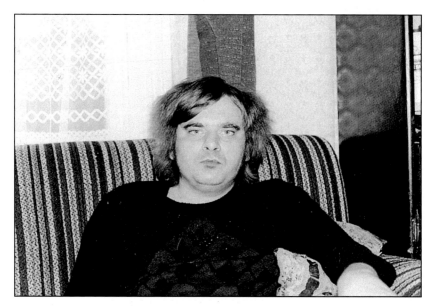

*Philip pictured at home after having been
diagnosed with schizophrenia*

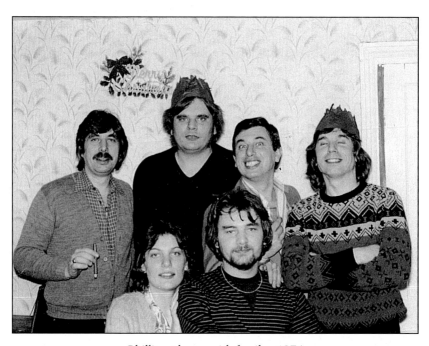

Phillip at home with family - 1974

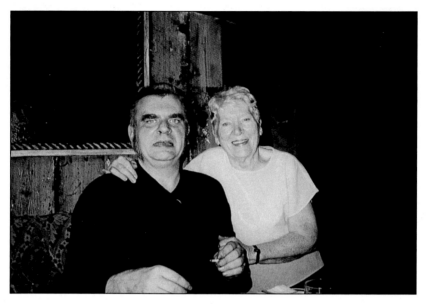

My mum with Philip. Always and ever caring

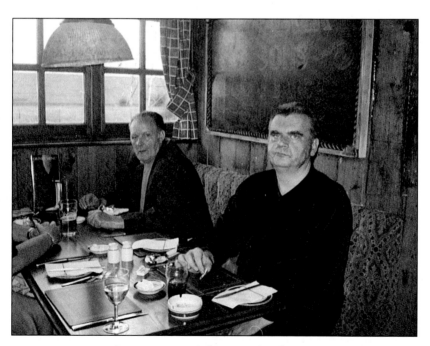

*Always a treat - Philip enjoys lunch, a pint
and smoke with his carers*

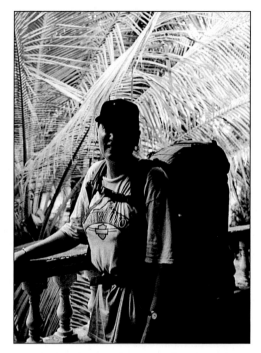

Sylvia backpacking in India - 1999

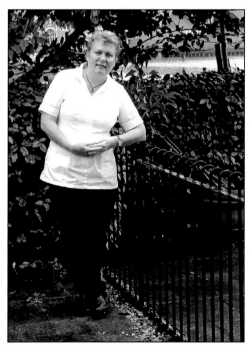

Sylvia as a student nurse Salford Quays - 2004

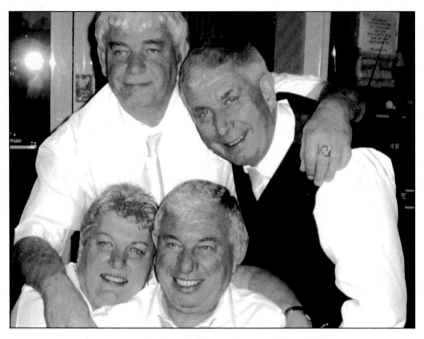

Paul, Alan, Sylvia and Ian – 2007

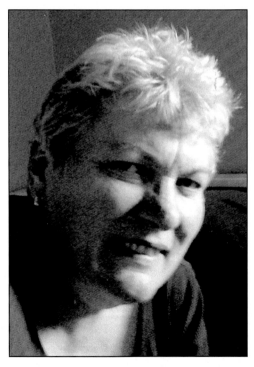

Sylvia present day

8

The Genetics of Deafness

There are an estimated nine million people in the United Kingdom with some degree of deafness. Most of them are elderly people with age-related hearing loss. It is thought that approximately 70,000 people use British Sign Language as their preferred language, many of them being from families with a long history of Deafness going back many generations. Referring to Deaf people with a capital 'D' designates them as members of a cultural and linguistic minority with their own distinct traditions and values.

Within most families communication flows freely and everyone joins in family discussions, conversations and banter. Our family was different - very different - as three of us were always at a loss to know what was being talked about. Other things that hearing people take for granted were also a mystery to us; for example, I remember going bird watching and egg collecting with Richard. As we budding 'twitchers' crept quietly through the bushes in the park, he grabbed hold of my arm saying, 'Sshhhh!! I can hear a bird singing!' I, of course, could hear nothing...

I was always curious to know how Philip, my twin brother Paul and I became deaf. When I was a teenager, aged about 13 or 14, I asked my mother why the three of us were deaf. She didn't have a clue and said that the doctor had never explained it to her. I checked whether we'd had any illnesses like meningitis but it seems there were none - certainly Mum didn't have any illnesses or viruses when she was pregnant. I was puzzled but left it there, just accepting that we'd been born deaf.

When I attended the Croydon College for the Access to Nursing course (2001-2002), I studied biology as one of the course modules. On one occasion the lecturer was talking about DNAShe talked about the cells in a person's body and how genealogy works. This was all very interesting to me and then it clicked in my mind. I realised that it was genetics that had caused the deafness in our family and that either my mother or father was carrying the deafness gene. Yet there seemed to be no history of deafness or any deafness present in their extended families or way back beyond. However and interestingly so, my mother later admitted that she had always been deaf in one ear and that she might have been the genetic carrier.

I became fascinated in the subject of DNA and genetics, taking every opportunity to study the subjects further. When I got the chance, I asked my lecturer if it could be that the three of us were deaf because of some genetic issue. She said this was certainly the case and I was relieved, that after years of speculation, my brothers and I finally knew the truth.

We all inherit characteristics, like the colour of our skin, eyes and hair, from our parents. It seems some forms or types of deafness can also be inherited. Every cell in our body has two copies of about 30,000 different genes - one copy is inherited from the mother and one from the father - and they are mostly grouped together in structures called chromosomes.

DNA is apparently built from four different chemical 'building blocks'. These blocks are strung together in a way that is unique to every gene and is known as the 'DNA sequence'. The DNA sequence of a single gene tells the cell how to make one of many thousands of proteins which the cell needs to be able to do its job. Sometimes the DNA sequence of a gene can change - this change is called a 'mutation' and these changes might mean that the gene won't function correctly. So, if the gene mutation interferes with the instructions for making the required protein needed for hearing, then it could cause deafness.

The chance of developing deafness through a mutated gene depends on whether the mutation is dominant or recessive. A dominant gene mutatio causes deafness when only one copy of the gene is affected. In this case, the affected gene can come from the mother or father with the chance of passing on this mutation to your children being one in two. However, dominant genes do not always have the same effect on everyone. Even in the same family, the gene can cause profound deafness in one person and mild deafness in another. Indeed sometimes, it might not affect a person's hearing at all.

A dominant gene mutation may have been in the family for generations. Alternatively, it can sometimes appear for the first time in a family without a prior history of deafness.

A recessive gene mutation causes deafness only when both copies of the gene are affected, so both the mother and father must both have passed on an affected gene. Someone who has a recessive mutation and a normal copy of the same gene will be hearing because the recessive gene 'recedes' into the background. They are called 'carriers' and can pass on the affected gene to their children. Most carriers never know they are carriers, unless they take a genetic test.

Recessive mutations are the most common cause of inherited deafness. A deaf person whose deafness is due to a recessive mutation, may have hearing parents and may also have deaf and hearing brothers and sisters with no previous family history of deafness, even though the deafness is genetic in origin.

When I learned all of this, I felt a huge burden lift from me. For years I had wondered why we were deaf and when people would question me, I would just shrug my shoulders. But now I know - it's all in the genes!

The Kenneth Family

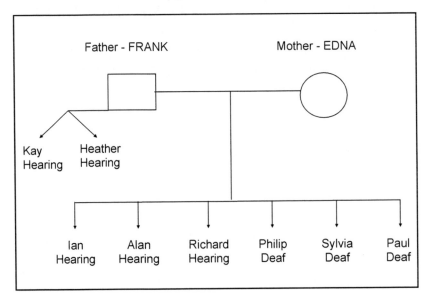

PART TWO

How My Brother
Developed Schizophrenia

9

Into Adulthood

From the age of 13 to 16, I was a typical teenager with a love of life and an innate curiosity about many things. I enjoyed hanging out with my school friends and the people that lived around us. I also started to experiment with things in life, like testing out religious beliefs, meeting different people and learning about their cultures, getting involved in sports, education and the environment.

With my brothers Philip and Paul, I was always out with a group of school friends going window shopping, out to the cinema or places of interest or just relaxing at school friends' homes. Occasionally, we would dare ourselves to do something different and head up to the lurid sex shops up in the West End. Here we'd have a laugh and learn something different! Puberty hit us with our bodies changing as we developed and matured. We became more aware of the physical and emotional differences between men and women.

The Saturday matinee at Stamford Hill was a regular for me, Paul and Philip. We loved the cartoons, feature films, westerns and thrillers. We would find the adventures of the

Lone Ranger thrilling with actors like Roy Rogers and Ronald Reagan. The cinema building was very old and it cost just a few pennies to get in for the afternoon session. Yet if Paul, Philip and I wanted to save money, one of us would pay for a single ticket and then sneak up to the back doors. We would then quietly let the others in under the gaze of the patrolling attendants! We would also make money by collecting empty Coca-Cola bottles and returning them to the confectionery shop. All those two-penny bits helped us build up a tidy sum!

Ian, Alan and Richard shared a passion for Ford cars. They bought a battered old blue Ford Zephyr and spent hours and hours reconditioning the engine, wire brushing the spark plugs, replacing the old bumpers with new chrome ones, repairing dents and re-upholstering the interiors. The front seat was a long bench seat that could fit four people. The car was cleaned out and washed weekly and the chrome polished to a deep shine. Our house often resembled a workshop as Ian, Alan and Richard worked on their cars, and those of their friends, outside in the street or in the garage at the back. Dad would get involved too, often pottering around to offer helpful advice or peering under the bonnet to tackle yet another mechanical problem.

Whilst this was going on, Paul and I were always busy at the local Deaf club in Green Lanes. I was focused on sports such as badminton, table tennis, darts and ladies football. This was all great fun but very time-consuming and it took up most of my teenage years! But I had some success and was selected to play for the Deaf Great Britain Netball Team throughout 1986-87 which was formed unofficially by the independent players of the English Netball Squad. The Deaf Great Britain Netball Team were invited to Australia to play in a tournament against Australia, New Zealand and Trinidad & Tobago but unfortunately were thrashed by the Australian team because of their years of experience. Since then the netball team has collapsed and so we never played in the Olympic Games. Paul did well at sport too and he enjoyed playing football at local club level.

Paul went on to marry a girl called Gillian and they had two children, Mark and Roxy. They were married for 13 years but later separated. Today the children live with their mother in Hertfordshire and Paul is regularly in touch with them. Paul himself now has a flat in Enfield which he shares with his partner, Karen.

Ian married Lillian in March 1968 and soon after, they emigrated to New Zealand on a cruise ship that took four weeks to arrive. Ian had the offer of a fantastic job as an engineer at Auckland Airport, but nevertheless, it was an emotional farewell for the family when the ship left Harwich docks. They later had two daughters, Angela and Judy, and lived there for 13 years before returning to England. Whilst the lifestyle appealed, Ian and Lillian eventually became homesick, missing their family and friends. But moving back to the UK wasn't without its issues. It was hard for Angela and Judy because they had to leave behind the many friends they had made at school.

Alan and Jackie also married in May of the same year. They lived nearby in Tottenham and eventually moved to Enfield. They bore three sons: Roy, Lee and James. Alan worked part-time for many years as a night security guard for Walthamstow dog racing stadium and also as a lorry driver. Jackie is an ambulance driver based at North Middlesex Hospital in North London.

Richard was seemingly in a world of his own. He and his wife Sue joined an Eastern-inspired religious cult that followed the spiritual guru known as the Maharaji. They had two daughters, Dawn and Zena. The whole family were devoted vegetarians and Richard and Sue followed the Maharaji wherever he went. As the influence of the Maharaji became stronger, they became more and more involved in the Divine Light Mission which followed the teachings of the teenage Maharaji. This seemingly attracted a large following which resulted in the Maharaji setting up his world headquarters in Denver, Colorado, where about a thousand young people filled the group's communes. The movement gradually declined after the Maharaji married his secretary, despite his mother's great protestations, and his family in India severed their connections with him.

Richard and his wife continued following the cult, but this came to an end when Sue had an affair with Richard's best friend who lived locally. Richard was left devastated with two very young daughters to look after. He came to live with us at our parents' house and I remember that at first he spent a lot of time in his bedroom. Gradually he began to recover emotionally and mentally. Soon after, he moved to Kent to bring up his two daughters and today it looks like a job well done. There is a strong father-daughter relationship and they remain close. Richard later went on to meet and fall in love with Michelle, with whom he had a daughter, Jasmine.

In person and to look at, Philip Kenneth was frighteningly handsome. Confident about his looks, he exuded a free-thinking, cool vibe. A lot of my female school friends liked him because he was a very good-looking young man, a typical blonde with deep blue eyes, gentle and quiet. He had an innocent charm that enabled him to get away with anything. He would carry a clean handkerchief to school every day and whenever he got the giggles, he would stifle the fits of laughter by pretending to blow his nose. Philip rarely got into trouble at school and was always respectful to the teachers. He was popular with his friends and he rubbed along well with just about everybody.

Whilst there were lots of girls who would hang around him at school, Philip kept his dignity and pride in himself. He liked to be independent, but would usually hang out with his best mate, Fred. They travelled to school together as Fred lived nearby. Many years later I was to chance upon Fred at

Finsbury Park station. We chatted about old times at school, pupils who had left, where they had gone and what they were doing. Some had got married, some had not and others had gone onto alternative lifestyles!

When we got onto the subject of Philip, I quietly said that he was mentally ill. Fred was stunned by this. He couldn't understand how Philip had developed his illness and he kept questioning himself as to how this had all come about. He asked if there was hope for his recovery. I explained that, sadly, this wasn't the case and that until a scientific cure is discovered, nothing would change.

After Ian, Alan, Richard and Paul had left home, Philip began truanting from school - sneaking back home to the house after Mum and Dad had left for work. They had absolutely no idea he'd been skipping school until they were notified that his absence record was appalling! In 1970, at the age of 15, Philip stopped going to school altogether and we started to become concerned for his mental well-being. He'd made a new friend called Tony and they seemed to spend most of their time experimenting with drugs. They would hang out with other friends in Hackney smoking cannabis and taking LSD, drugs that gave them a disturbed sense of reality.

10

Tony

Having left school with no CSE or GCE qualifications, Philip had no sense of direction and he regressed to become a resentful, sullen and moody teenager. The school authorities tried to get Philip to continue his education but to no avail. So did Mum and Dad but they had even less luck with him. During this time, Philip made little effort to speak to anyone and kept himself to himself. In his self-imposed isolation, he just stayed in his bedroom for most of the time. I had no idea how desperately out of control he was about to become.

Philip became more and more involved with his friend Tony. A hearing boy who lived locally, he was gaunt and thin with jet-black hair and was always dressed in casual clothes. We didn't really know who he was or where he'd sprung from. He lived about a mile away, we thought, and spent a lot of time on the doorstep of my parents' house whispering or making secret plans with Philip. Mum and Dad didn't like this at all - they were fearful and suspicious of him; he behaved strangely and was most uncooperative.

One day, I went up to Philip's bedroom to tell him that

dinner was ready. I caught him sitting on his bed preparing a cannabis smoke in tobacco paper. The room smelt funny and odd, but as Philip hadn't seen me come in, I tiptoed away quietly. Feeling shocked and terrified at what I'd seen, as I'd never encountered such things before, I stuttered and blurted it all out to Dad. He was shocked and couldn't believe it. He confronted Philip who obviously denied it and raged that it was up to him what he wanted to do in his own bedroom. I was thinking, 'Drugs … what the hell was he doing with drugs!?' I kept asking myself over and over, 'Why is Philip using drugs? Is he unhappy? Has he lost respect for us?'

Clearly Philip was under the influence of Tony, such that all he could think about was cannabis and LSD. Deep into drugs, the white LSD tablets were all that mattered to him.

Whilst all this was going on, an old school friend of mine, Yvonne Clarke, took a fancy to Philip. Yvonne was quite a character - a strong cockney woman born and raised on the Isle of Dogs in East London. It was Yvonne who introduced me to the famous East ender's staple, pie 'n' mash. We would regularly frequent the Pie and Mash cafe in Chrisp Street where we would natter long and hard over mugs of steaming tea!

Yet on their first date together and with an excited Yvonne at his side, Philip called in on Tony. Yvonne couldn't quite understand this and felt quite left out as the two of them discussed their 'underworld' business. Having had enough, Yvonne asked Philip if they could leave whereupon Tony promptly made it clear she should go off alone.

Stunned and shocked, Yvonne left and went home really upset. She never believed Philip would choose his mate over her. Sadly, at the time none of us knew any of this and it was only many years later that we learnt what had gone on. Tony's grip on Philip was increasing and every day they would be hanging out together. We never knew where they went or what they did, but increasingly, Philip would come home looking stoned and behaving strangely, laughing at the smallest things. His eyes were glazed red and his pupils large, looking dark and menacing. He stank of cannabis and became a total stranger to us, becoming ever more impenetrable.

Mum was hurt, lost, grief-stricken almost. I could see that she just didn't know what to do. Once I even saw her staring at Philip's photo, lamenting the little boy lost ... but there was nothing I could say to make her feel better. We were all struggling to deal with it.

A few months after that, Philip became more and more alienated, isolating himself further from the family and continuing to develop his close friendship with Tony. The paraphernalia of drugs littered his bedroom and no amount of cajoling, shouting or crying would make him see any different. He wasn't going to give up and, hooked on cannabis and LSD, Philip was now an addict.

Keeping Tony away became more and more difficult. My parents tried to ward him off when he appeared at the doorstep, but he always found a way of getting through to Philip. But then Philip became seriously ill and he was unable to function or communicate properly. He spent most of his time in his bedroom being quiet and sleeping. He slept during the day but would then be awake at night when he would just stare at the television till nothing was on. Dad would often go to Philip's room early in the morning to tell him to stop walking around and to turn off the television which would blare out for hours on end...

It was at about this time that relations between Philip and Tony soured. There was no explanation from Philip as to what had happened but Tony stopped coming round. At one point Tony tried to get back some money which he said Philip owed for drugs, but Mum and Dad threatened him with the police. Maybe it was this, but I always saw him as a coward who knew that Philip's mental health had deteriorated and yet he did nothing to help - nothing at all.

Locally, it was common knowledge that Tony was a drug dealer who'd been supplying drugs to teenagers. Neighbours and friends knew what he was up to and even told my Mum and Dad so, but they were powerless. Connected to other drug dealers as he was, he was all-powerful, all-pervasive and there was nothing anyone could do to stop him. Tony had an invisible grip over Philip and he manipulated him no end, making him dependant, wanton. Philip was vulnerable and easily influenced - Tony knew this and used his power to control him.

With Tony gone, we were left to pick up the shattered pieces. Tony had ruined Philip's mental health and we were left not knowing what to do. My parents didn't know who to turn to or where they could get help. The irreparable damage had been done and I'm absolutely sure that if Philip hadn't have met Tony, things would have been so different and he would have had a better life.

11

Philip's Illness

P hilip's illness became worse. He started to hallucinate and respond to voices in his head. He stayed at home every day and refused to go out socially or to try and find a job, no matter how menial. Whenever he did get a job, he would last just a couple of days. He would say that the people at work didn't want him because his behaviour was erratic and odd. One of his managers from work approached my parents to say that Philip was mentally unwell and not fit for the workplace. We were devastated to hear this and yet things went from bad to worse. He became increasingly aggressive and reclusive, often not bothering to get up in the morning. The more we tried to show our concern and support him the more negative and evasive he became. We would ask him what was wrong and he'd just say, 'I don't know' or he would gaze into the middle distance and shrug his shoulders. Philip had no idea what was wrong with him and, as one would expect, didn't realise he had a mental illness.

Philip existed in a world of his own, often talking or mumbling random thoughts to himself, before then laughing or shouting for no apparent reason. He had emotional responses that were back to front and inappropriate to his surroundings; for example, he would laugh at sad news or appear unconcerned by important occurrences. I remember once when watching a TV programme that was about some real-life tragedy, Philip just sat and laughed. Another time, when he was watching a funny programme, he sat morose and glum. I wondered if Philip was aware of how he was reacting as he became preoccupied with issues that appeared abstract and bizarre to those around him.

There were many times when Philip expressed paranoid ideas or visibly reacted to the hallucinations he experienced. These hallucinations usually took the form of hearing 'voices' as is common in people experiencing schizophrenia. With Philip, the voices would chide his behaviour and sometimes order him to do things. I used to dread this and I could tell when it was happening. Philip would start shouting 'Fuck off' loudly. Or it would be, 'I don't want you', 'Go away' or 'Go to hell and fuck you!!'

All of this was awful to see and I used to wonder what on earth Philip was seeing or who it was he was talking to; did the voices come from somewhere in the room or somewhere outside? Did Philip think the voices were real and were they whispering or shouting at him? Did this happen most days or just the odd few days?

It was the strange stare that gave it away. When his face went white and blank I knew he was hallucinating; there was nothing behind his eyes, they were vacant, empty, macabre almost. At first, it was hurtful to hear the unpleasant outbursts but we all knew that it wasn't the Philip we knew. We became used to him shouting and would tell him to be quiet. Every day he swore, ranted and abused us. Every day we told him to shut up or go to his room. Every day it got worse … and whilst I wanted to empathise with him, I just couldn't.

There were times when as well as shouting, Philip would converse with a non-existent person. He would hold these strange and bizarre conversations and you would think the other person was in the room. Sometimes he would be laughing at the other person, sometimes shouting and it all sounded utterly convincing. But then for Philip I'm sure it was, as his perception of the world was now very different to that of ours.

My family were naturally embarrassed by Philip. They struggled to cope with the swearing and verbal abuse. My parents were strict and respectable - swearing wasn't for them, they thought it rude and offensive. Whenever we had visitors, Philip, on cue, would start shouting at them. He would be despatched to his room sharpish but we knew people were uncomfortable and slowly but surely, they began to stop calling and visiting ... they didn't know what to say or what to do. Plus of course they didn't want their own children to witness this spectacle and were worried that Philip would do something even more bizarre, that his behaviour would become physically violent.

Reflecting on an article I read some time ago, many friends and family members of people with schizophrenia report knowing early on that something was wrong with their loved one, but they just don't understand what's going on or what to do. Other people may notice a change in the person's behaviour, or in the content of their speech. My family and I recognised these problems and we discussed long and hard how to deal with it. Eventually, my mother realised Philip had serious problems and so she arranged for the GP to assess him. Immediately the GP referred Philip to Dr John Denmark, a psychiatrist at Prestwich Hospital, Manchester. It was in 1972 that, accompanied by my mother, Philip was diagnosed as suffering from paranoid schizophrenia. We were heartbroken and relieved in equal measure.

A pioneer in his field, Dr John Denmark was an honorary consultant psychiatrist at the John Denmark Unit, Mental

Health Services of Salford NHS Trust (formerly Prestwich Hospital). He was the first psychiatrist to develop dedicated psychiatric services for Deaf people and the only psychiatrist at that time to properly assess Deaf patients who were in need of care. Dr Denmark's book entitled *Deafness and Mental Health*, published in 1994, was a seminal work and a landmark publication. His knowledge of general psychiatry and general medicine was extensive, and he was much sought after, even in his retirement, to provide independent reports for mental health review tribunals and other such bodies.

Devastated, my Mum drew upon her inner strengths to support Philip, liaising with Dr Denmark over treatment strategies. In assessing Philip, Dr Denmark also assessed the wider family. He found no family history of anyone being diagnosed with mental illness or schizophrenia, only Philip. I was convinced that Philip's medical condition had been triggered by his use of cannabis resin and LSD. I thought maybe there was a genetic link somewhere but we discounted this because if a faulty gene is present, there is a one in four chance the person will have the condition.

So now we all knew - Philip was suffering from a mental illness and had been diagnosed with paranoid schizophrenia. I think what shocked both family and friends was that Philip himself didn't realise the impact of the illness that was destroying him. But from the moment he was correctly diagnosed by Dr Denmark, he began to slowly and gradually stop functioning. This was just awful for us and we moved closely around Philip to support and care for him as best we could. But we'd had no formal training in mental health or schizophrenia and, for the most of the time, we were helpless.

When need - or should I say exasperation - arose, we would get advice from the GP and Dr Denmark. We also got help from two voluntary organisations, SANE and MIND. Both these organisations were established to help make a difference to the lives of those affected by mental illness. My parents were hugely grateful for the support they received, as it helped them determine strategies for dealing with Philip's illness and enabled them to get a sense of where they stood with the health service and local authority, what care Philip was entitled to and where it could be obtained.

Philip had never ever described his feelings towards becoming mentally ill. If anything it seemed he was losing the ability to articulate his thoughts, fears and concerns. Every day, more and more, he further lost control as someone or something continued to take over him. His thoughts and emotions were being driven by some implanted force and as a result, he became less and less communicative. His energy sapped away, his zest for life eroded and his concentration became minimal. It became ever harder for Philip to describe his feelings to us and we had to always second guess what he was thinking about and what it was he wanted us to do.

It would have been different if Philip was able to communicate with us - to tell us what was going in his mind and how he was feeling. But this didn't seem to happen. We could never tell if he having flashbacks because of his illness or if he was afraid, for example, of the dark. Was he hoping for another outcome or had he abandoned his dreams, prospects and aspirations? Did he realise he'd been robbed of his youth or was he unaware? Did something on television trigger his paranoia or did his fear originate elsewhere? We just never knew and the more all this went on, the more upset we all became. But for Philip we had no choice, we had to pull together to support him, to be strong and to be united. If nothing more, this was the least we could do.

12

Affecting the Family

Yet from the darkness we descended to the depths ... Philip's symptoms worsened and he was constantly shouting and hollering. At all times of the day and night he would scream and swear away. He looked as if he was being persecuted and that something was possessing him. It was frightening to be in a room with him, the atmosphere and tension was just unbearable.

Philip was never up early in the morning. He would emerge at lunchtime and the atmosphere would change instantly. He would expect that Mum had made lunch for him or if there was none forthcoming, then he would ask her to make some. Often she would leave her unfinished meal to organise whatever it was he wanted. Dad would just ignore Philip and mutter under his breath to himself. Sometimes he would immerse himself in a TV programme or go out to the pub, anything to just get away from Philip and the tension he created. Whenever Philip was in the lounge I felt nervous and was unable to relax, I was always on edge and had a feeling of dread in the pit of my stomach. Day after day this feeling went on and I hated the situation we were in, especially as Philip was becoming increasingly and dangerously manic.

Philip's aggression began to know no bounds and he often had to be restrained by my Dad, my brothers and myself. None of us liked what we were doing to Philip but it had to be done. On one occasion, Philip saw Mum holding a purse and he tried to strangle her to get money for booze and cigarettes. Quickly recovering from our shock, Paul and I had to fight him off. Mum was shocked too - terrified - but she bottled it up, she didn't want to talk about it. But this went on and on; time and time again Philip would threaten Mum with a kitchen knife for money. He was becoming increasingly dependent upon drink and cigarettes and had developed a strong craving for cider because it was cheap and easy to get drunk on. That's all Philip was interested in - alcohol and tobacco. Mum received a carer's allowance which was supposed to pay for Philip's food, clothes and other needs, but he saw this as his 'beer money' to be used as he wished.

There was no getting away from the fact that Philip was becoming dangerous and we now had to hide away sharp kitchen knives for safety reasons. I remember one argument when yet again Philip was again trying to get money off Mum. Paul and I were trying to help her and there was lots of shuffling and pushing about. We pushed Philip hard away and with a 'Crack!' his elbow smashed the window, shattering glass on the pavement below. Hearing the noise, our next-door neighbour, Rita, scurried round to see what all the wondering what was going on. To add our embarrassment the police were called. Philip was given a caution from the police who, regretfully, were to become closely acquainted with my brother. Dad came home from work and was furious to hear what had happened; he obviously had to buy a window pane and replace the broken window.

Philip would go to great lengths to steal anything. He

stole any money that we left around the house or in our bedrooms. On many an occasion he was cautioned by the police for stealing alcohol from the local off-licence. Yet the police wouldn't charge him because of his mental state and because he wasn't fit to plead. The frequent visits by the police became the talk of the neighbourhood, such that people would stop Mum in the street and ask if everything was ok. The shame and pain we felt was immeasurable ... police cars were a regular sight on our doorstep and over time, the police got to know us. I wouldn't have said they were sympathetic but they began to talk to us in a familiar, friendly way.

Philip would sleep irregularly, staying awake late into the night and arising groggily in the afternoons. When he was up late, he would nurse and drink a one-litre bottle of cider. He would drink till he was sick and then we would have to clean up the mess. Time and time again, Mum and I had to clean up vomit and all the other detritus discarded by Philip. The disgust we felt was paramount and all-consuming.

If Philip made himself a cup of tea, he would splash in about five lumps of sugar and spill the scalding sticky liquid everywhere. He'd never, ever clean himself or the mess he made up. His living skills and his self-awareness were non-existent and he had no enthusiasm for cooking, cleaning or washing anything. He was slowly but surely ruining the house with his spillages, cigarette burns and general abandonment. We had to buy tiled carpets so that damaged carpet could be easily replaced and I was always worried Philip would be careless in the kitchen or with a cigarette and start a devastating house fire. If none of us were at home, he would simply eat cold baked beans straight from the tin and make himself toast. Not surprisingly, with this poor dietary intake, Philip developed type two diabetes a few years later - the effect of too much sugar in his tea and too much cider. Sometimes when I buy alcohol in the supermarket and see cider, it reminds me of

Philip. The sweet, sickly smell of the stuff makes me nauseous to this day.

The incessant arguments, fights and the need to restrain Philip were taking an ever-increasing toll on the family. Every day, he was ranting, shouting and raving at the auditory hallucinations his drug and alcohol-induced psychosis was causing. In one episode Philip picked up a kitchen knife and ran amok through the house. We were terrified of him and now we had to call the police for help. He was too out of control, too big, too violent for us to manage. This happened time and time again, with soul-destroying and heart-breaking regularity.

One particular fight saw Dad having to restrain Philip on the floor. In the heat of the moment, through frustration and anger, Dad just lost it and Philip ended up with a black eye. This quite simply frightened and upset all of us. Mum was angry with Dad about Philip's black eye and the tension was terrible, just terrible. Dad had to go out for a couple of hours just to calm down and we all had to be quiet when he returned home ... he was in a foul mood, in a dark place. Another day, another argument saw Philip stab Paul's earlobe with a brass poker. There was an argument over a paraffin stove which Philip kept for himself in his room. Philip attacked Paul during the argument, who then needed hospital treatment and stitches.

I found myself constantly wondering what was happening to us - what was going to happen next? To what depths would we descend?

Perhaps it was this ... Philip became a voyeur. He pierced the door of the bathroom with a screwdriver so he could peep through. He even pierced my bedroom door and I had to cover the holes by hanging my bathrobe up. The damage was such that later Dad filled up the holes with Polyfilla and repainted the door. When he couldn't use the door to peer, Philip chose to stare from Mum and Dads' bedroom window, where he would watch me having a bath. From that point on I always checked that the bathroom windows were lowered and that no one could see in. But what was Philip thinking when he made the holes? Was he thinking I was just some unknown female and not his sister? Did he not have any consideration for me? Even now I'm a little paranoid when I am having a bath, I always keep an eye on the door, making sure there is no one there peeping through. I never realised it at the time, but all this still affects me today. I can never now properly enjoy a bath and have to use aromatic candles to help me relax.

One night, I awoke from a deep sleep when I felt something wasn't quite right. As I came to, I realised Philip was above me, fondling my breasts. I thought I was dreaming but when I realised what was happening I screamed, 'Daaaaaaaaad!!!', 'Daaaaaaaaad!!!' Startled as he was, Philip took fright and ran out the room just as Dad arrived to see what all the commotion was. When I told him what Philip had been doing he was stunned - just stunned. He couldn't believe it. In a white rage and livid with anger, Dad told Philip never to touch me again. But he did - several times.

I began to think I was losing it - I just couldn't handle Philip's behaviour any more, not least because it was disturbing my sleep pattern as I would lie awake fearful that he was going to come in. Night after night, I would creep past his bedroom door to get to my room. Then once in bed I would cry myself to sleep as I couldn't bear it any more. This couldn't go on, so Dad put a Yale lock on my bedroom door. But whilst this fixed the door, I now felt like a prisoner in my own room. This was madness I thought, carrying a key around the house and staying up in my room to avoid Philip if my parents were out. But whilst I was able to sleep properly now, I was still in fear of Philip. Sometimes I would go to bed with Polly our dog acting as a guard dog - she would enjoy the relief from being hassled by Philip and would sprawl herself across the bed next to me.

We were now at a point where I couldn't stay in the house alone with Philip. He was so unpredictable and I never knew if he would be exposing himself or up to some other trouble. I felt intense fear all the time when living at Bethune Road. Nowadays, I rarely have nightmares about Philip, but there are times when I wake up drenched in sweat, reliving the agony of past incidents. All of this was impacting upon Mum and Dad too. They would argue over what he was doing and there were times when they wouldn't be talking to each other. Mum was naturally protective of Philip, whilst Dad was protective of me. This in itself helped create a lingering tension.

At the age of 17, I had my first serious relationship with a boy. I spent many weekends at his house in Streatham and sometimes we went off to the St John of Beverley Club for the Deaf, in Green Lanes, to play games and sport. All of this was aimed at getting me away from home three or four times a week. I also used to escape from Bethune Road by visiting the local library. There I would take my time to read the books and magazines, pondering what I was going to do with my life. I found the library a very relaxing place to be and I eagerly read volume upon volume; my favourite books being *The Lion, The Witch and The Wardrobe* and the books about the mischievous cat with the red and white hat - *The Cat in The Hat* by Dr Seuss. At the library I felt safe, I was able to concentrate on things and be myself. There wasn't the constant threat of arguments and violence. I still use libraries today and it was in Beckenham library that I wrote much of this book.

There were times when I also took comfort from our dog Polly. She was never comfortable or settled when Philip was around. In fact she was terrified of him and would cower under the dining table or hide if he was about. Her legs would shake with fear when he called her. He would often want to stroke her fur and at times he would lift up Polly's two front legs and hug her. She hated this and would yelp to get away. But Philip couldn't be told to stop - it would just inflame him more.

There was also the time Philip lost Polly. He took her to Edmonton to visit our Auntie Glad. He took the bus there, which was fine, but on the journey home, the driver refused to allow Polly on. So Philip simply got on the bus and left the dog behind. We were, of course, out of our minds with worry when he arrived at the house with no dog! But about four hours later, we heard Polly barking away - miraculously she had found her way home, having trotted for five miles along traffic-filled roads and noisy streets. We were amazed and relieved; I was just so pleased to see her and rewarded her with a huge mountain of treats!

But back at home, things were coming to a head. The situation with Philip was draining us all and I could see that my parents couldn't cope. They could see this too and so they pleaded with the GP, Dr Freeman, for help. Perhaps he didn't know what to expect, but when he arrived at the house he was shocked by Philip's mental state and appearance. His condition had visibly worsened and he recommended that a social worker visit to assess Philip as soon as possible. When the social worker eventually arrived, Philip was in no condition to talk as he was hallucinating and swearing. It was impossible for the terrified social worker who had no way of assessing Philip under the circumstances. Whilst he could see what we were all dealing with, there was little he could do at the time.

We were now at a point where the problems were becoming insurmountable. Fights were a daily occurrence and we were becoming drained. Dad contacted Social Services again and specifically asked for a social worker for the Deaf. Eventually we received a visit and after much questioning, discussion and deliberation, it was proposed that Philip should be sectioned. But Mum refused to agree to this and insisted she would look after Philip at home. This naturally led to more and more arguments with Mum trying to protect him, whilst Dad was ever at a loss with Philip's moods and tempers.

It must have been so hard for Mum trying to protect Philip from the family and the public. He was her son, whom she had borne and raised; I can empathise with her feelings and yet I also understand how Dad felt. Mum faced a lot of criticism from both the family and friends for not having Philip sectioned, but I could see it had taken its toll on her too. I felt torn between Mum and Dad, but I couldn't take either side because I knew how they both, differently, felt about Philip's illness.

Community care hadn't been of much use to us. Although it was aimed at providing full support for people with mental illness living at home, we received little of tangible benefit. We expected some involvement in agreeing what care or treatment would be offered but there was nothing forthcoming, no protection from abuse, help with finances or legal support.

For Mum there was another, deeper, dimension to Philip's illness. She believed all Philip's woes stemmed from an Ouija board game way back which had upset her. She'd been playing with two of her sisters and some friends, when some communication was made and suddenly the glass flew off the table with a crash. For reasons unknown, Mum blamed herself for this and believed the punishment she received was Philip's illness; I'm not at all convinced by this. My brothers and I actually suspected that my mother had had a brief affair when she was at Maynards. Perhaps this was why she was being 'punished'? Philip's appearance wasn't much different from ours but he had blond hair and blue eyes, whereas the rest of us all had brown or black hair. Why an affair may have happened and exactly with whom, we'll never know. My parents kept themselves to themselves and rarely involved us with in any of their problems. Maybe because my Dad was working literally every day and night to keep the family together, Mum went astray? Was it the affair and Mum having to work at two jobs a day that upset Dad and led to his heart problems? Again, we'll never know.

As Philip's decline progressed, he became more unwashed, unshaven and dirty. He would forget to clean his teeth and his personal hygiene just fell apart. He stank and his hair was messy and uncombed. Philip refused to go to the hairdressers and would cut his hair himself, though sometimes he would ask Mum to help him. As a result his eyebrows and sideburns grew longer and wider, giving him a wild, unkempt look. Philip wore the same jumper every day and rarely changed his clothes. It was obvious he'd lost any awareness of how he looked or how he carried himself. He would have food and cider stains all down his front. His comprehension appeared to be going and he was finding it hard to concentrate on reading or watching the television. Philip had become unrecognisable to the family and when Mum's relatives came to visit they were appalled. Ian's children, his two daughters Angela and Judy, and Alan's children, his three sons Roy, Lee and James, nicknamed Philip 'the Hulk'. Standing at 6 feet 2 inches tall, unkempt and wild, he really did look a Marvel comic horror. Ian and Alan, unfortunately and sadly, adopted and used the name continually. They threatened their children that if they ever took drugs then this would be the result. It seemed to me that the message hit home so perhaps some perverse good was derived from this tragedy.

One night, I got home from work and I settled down to watch the television news   whilst Mum prepared the dinner. Whatever was being reported captured my interest and Philip could see this, so he suddenly got up, turned the television off and then sat down again. Furious, I got up to turn the television back on again and Philip moved to turn it off. Very quickly we were in an argument and then a full blown fight. Mum and my sister-in-law tried to intervene but I told them to stay away as my cardigan was ripped, my tooth chipped and my face scratched.

This was it. I'd had enough and so I walked out of the family home, my home...

With nowhere to go I turned up at my friend Jackie's to calm myself down. No one knew I was there so Mum and Dad were going frantic with worry but I needed to get away. Deep into the night and over the following days I talked to Jackie and poured out all my feelings and frustrations. I was angry that I'd had to live with all the fear caused by Philip. I was angry that Mum wouldn't accept professional help and that she kept taking responsibility for Philip's actions. I was so angry, just so angry.

Eventually Mum and Dad begged me to come home because they couldn't handle the situation. It had all become so difficult for them. I compromised and agreed that I'd return so long as they got Philip referred for professional help. At long last they agreed to this, but in reality they had no choice. Things with Philip were going from very, very bad to very much worse.

Philip continued to respond and react to auditory hallucinations. He was caught quite a few times exposing himself to women in public places and as a result was arrested by the police. On some occasions he would spend the night in the cells. Yet, as before, he couldn't be charged as he was classified as mentally ill. He even exposed himself to family members such as my niece Angela, who was just a young teenager, and neighbours like the Burns family. He would stand in his bedroom window masturbating to get Carol's attention - something Dad put a stop to by nailing the window shut. Obviously the police would be called and, yet again, we'd have to suffer the agony of shame and embarrassment. Mum and Dad had to profusely apologise to the Burns family, but they were sympathetic and never sought to cause us any problems.

One day Philip went to visit Alan in Tottenham but he wasn't in. There was only Jackie at home who was busy cutting up materials to make something or other. Without any word or hint of warning, Philip dropped his trousers in front of her. Jackie was furious and, holding up a pair of scissors, threatened him to stop; it worked because he left and ran off in a hurry, knowing that Jackie was not afraid of him. Alan was livid, but what could we do? There was one option and it was now looking more and more inevitable...

13

Admission to Hospital

With Philip out of control, Dad finally managed to persuade Mum to contact Dr Freeman and the social worker for help. Again, they attended at the house to assess Philip's mental state and this time there was no dispute, Philip needed medical treatment. Eventually he was sectioned and the police arrived at our home to collect him. Accompanied by a psychiatrist and staff nurse, he was admitted to St Clements Psychiatric Hospital in Bow Road. He was detained there for six months under Section 3 of the Mental Health Act 1983.

Mum regularly visited Philip at the hospital as she knew that somewhere inside his mind was the boy she loved, gorgeous and quiet. She was constantly asking herself, 'Why did it have to happen to Philip?' Unfamiliar with the practice and principles of the mental health system, she was - at first - unhappy with the way Philip was treated. But as she got to know the staff and after several long conversations with the psychiatrist, she realised that it was the best place for Philip.

On one occasion when Mum and I went to see Philip she was quite overcome. Drawing upon her maternal love she said, 'Philip, I am worried about you and I can see that you are suffering deeply. I know that the professionals at this hospital have been busy observing you, treating your symptoms, and trying to rehabilitate you'. She went on, 'You are angry because you have been diagnosed with a mental illness. You feel angry because all your friends are doing normal things like going to school, going out on dates and having fun'. Philip fixed us with us with his blue eyes; 'Why me?' he said. 'Why has this happened to me?' We couldn't answer that - we didn't have an answer and so left in despair before the pain totally engulfed us.

I always found visiting Philip a nightmare, a living nightmare. We would travel by the 106 bus from where we lived to Mile End station. From there it was a short walk to the hospital. Shaking and scared - the word 'mental' always put a fear into my mind that I would never get out - I would enter the ward, its brightly whitewashed walls contrasting sharply with the wooden doors and dark coloured floors. I would feel the tension rising up inside me and the other patients frightened me. There was always one particular woman who would be walking around in circles mumbling to herself and unaware of her surroundings. That was the moment it hit me ... when I realised that it wasn't just Philip who was mentally ill, but others too. It was awkward and embarrassing to see other patients in the ward and how they behaved, but I gradually began to learn that they couldn't control their behaviour. It wasn't their fault they were there - it was the illness they were suffering.

We would constantly ask Philip how he was getting on in the ward. He would say that he wasn't happy being away from home because he missed the comforts of home and family. Philip would frequently become tearful, but he would never say much as he didn't quite know what to say. As he didn't know any of the other patients he was very much alone, isolated by his Deafness and tortured by his illness. Mum and I were heartbroken but there was little we could do.

To tackle his illness, Philip underwent Electro-Convulsive Therapy (ECT) where electrodes were attached to his temples and electrical currents passed through the brain. This kind of therapy is a psychiatric treatment which has been used in mental health hospitals for many years. The patient should receive a muscle relaxant and is then anaesthetised to ensure that there is no pain. The electrodes are placed on either side of the temples and an electrical current is run across the brain. ECT aims to stimulate the brain so that it responds better to neuro-transmitters. Whilst it is a therapy that has some benefit, it can also have some side effects. Mum for sure wasn't comfortable with the thought of ECT treatment and couldn't bear the notion of Philip having electricity shot through his brain. I would find myself pondering all that Philip was going through and how both his moods and mind changed, of the neuroses, fears, troubles and poor concentration he endured whilst the rest of us lived 'normal' lives.

The problem with visits was that Philip would want to come home with us. There was one day when he was in a very bad mood and he insisted he was going home. We would try and reassure him he was in the best place for care and treatment but to no avail. Then he started to get upset, to shout and push. Eventually the nurses came along and asked Philip to calm down as he was distressing the other patients. As hard as it was, we had no choice, we had to leave, but I found the whole thing very upsetting and I felt for Philip.

A few months later, Philip was discharged from the hospital and his mental state improved with medication. He also received a 'depot injection' which was given every four weeks by the community psychiatric nurse. This was a preparation of some solution which was injected into the buttock area and which would then release into the body over a period of weeks. In addition, Philip had to have anti-psychotic medications which alleviated the symptoms of schizophrenia. But there were downsides - Philip's weight increased, he showed signs of tremor and he became quite restless, blinking or rolling his eyes frequently in a strange manner. After a few years of receiving medication through this method, Philip was prescribed an alternative medication for his schizophrenia called Olanzapine.

When Philip was sectioned, he never showed any insight or feelings of what was going on. As a schizophrenic, he may have recognised the existence of his illness but never brought the subject of this up with the family.

I understand that people respond differently to anti-psychotic medication and that sometimes, several different drugs must be tried before the right one is found which controls the symptoms best and has the least side effects.

After Philip was discharged from hospital, I realised that it was time for me to move out. I couldn't cope with living with him any more as he made me fearful and nervous. I informed my parents, bought a one-bedroom flat over in Forest Gate and moved in. I'd simply had enough of Philip after 13 years living under the same roof and wasn't prepared to take the mental or emotional stress any more. Mum and Dad were struggling too ... they were getting older and were less and less able to manage him. As Philip was now back at home they would dread the sound of the telephone ringing, thinking it would be the police on the case of his latest misdemeanour; had he exposed himself again or had he tried to raid an off-licence for alcohol? Whatever was it now? It was almost impossible to convey the sense of dread hanging over my parents.

Mum and Dad felt it was time for Philip to be properly looked after and they applied to have him taken into care. This was a momentous and difficult decision that saw Philip assessed and placed in the Clapton Common Residential Home for the Mentally Ill. Here he was settled and a treatment strategy determined. Under medication, his mental state remained stable and he received therapeutic care from the nurses. Philip spent a long time at this home and he was able to interact with the other residents. There were day trips to the seaside, places of local interest, ten pin bowling evenings and visits to the cinema. All in all, he had a reasonable quality of life.

It was at about this time that Ian and Lillian returned home from New Zealand. They had been away for 13 years and whilst pleased to see them I couldn't contain my anger. I took a view that Ian let us down, that he had neglected us and that he had no idea of what we'd been going through. Mum had certainly tried to keep Ian and Lillian informed of what was occurring, but there is only so much that letters can say and I wasn't sure Ian had really understood the gravity of the situation. But when Ian went to see Philip there was no doubt … he was shocked to see the state of him and how he changed from a good-looking young chap to this obese, older man. Ian was mortified by what he saw and wept uncontrollably.

Eventually Mum and Dad moved to a house in Enfield to be near my three brothers. They didn't tell Philip where they were because they feared for their safety and they also wanted to live out their retirement quietly. Mum was torn between Philip and the family and although she knew she'd done the right thing having sent him to a care home, it still hurt. Ever faithful to her son, she would regularly phone Philip and visited every fortnight. She never, ever gave up on him.

Once I'd moved to the flat I had no desire to see Philip again. I wanted to put him out of my mind and forget all the traumas he'd caused. It must have been about five years later that I realised it wasn't entirely his fault that he had become mentally ill. Over time, I came to terms with this and decided to put aside my feelings aside. I contacted the care home where Philip was residing. Part of me was curious and I wanted to see how he had changed and what had been happening to him. I spoke to one of the carers there for almost two hours. I was in tears and all over the place, talking about the past and how it had affected me and the family. The carer listened patiently and understood how I felt when I explained the anger and grief Philip's illness had caused us. I poured out more and more and as I did so, I realised that I hadn't actually discussed Philip with anyone for years. It had all been too painful. I actually found the call quite helpful and decided that I would keep in touch with the carer. She understood how I felt and was very sympathetic. She enabled me to express my feelings and kept me informed of Philip's progress at the home, making the point that the staff and other healthcare professionals were grateful Mum and I kept in touch with them about Philip.

Unburdening to the carer helped me open up and discuss matters with other people too. I poured out everything to my close friend Niki Roeder who was most supportive. But at least now I was able to do this - previously I had suffered in silence, in tears for myself and my family too.

It was unfortunate that Philip's mental illness was caused by street drugs. I don't know whether these drugs can trigger off long-term mental illness on their own, but it is possible that Philip was vulnerable. There is certainly evidence that the use of cannabis doubles the risk of developing schizophrenia. We who have lived with the consequences of cannabis and other drugs know only too well that it destroys lives, families and communities.

14

Philip's Death

last saw Philip when Mum asked me to go with her to tell
him that Dad had died. This was December 1994 and I was
resistant given that I hadn't seen Philip for five years. I felt
nothing but hatred for him, for all that he done to the family
and for the total lack of remorse he showed. I was also scared
that he would attack me. However, I couldn't let Mum go alone
and so, reluctantly, I agreed to join her.

When we reached the residential care home in Clapton
Common, my heart started to pump and I felt my pulse racing.
Clammy with fear, I began to feel hot, ill. Mum sensed this and
sought to reassure me, talking to me calmly to allay my fears. I
explained to Mum that all the years of trauma, upset and pain
just wouldn't go away and she understood. She said we'd all
suffered but that we needed to 'move on'.

As we waited in the reception area, Philip appeared. He
said 'Hello' and stared at me for a while. I just sat there
quietly thinking Philip probably thought he would never see
me again. He asked if we would like to have cup of tea and
he went on to make us a sticky, sugary concoction. Although

it tasted too sweet, I didn't want to complain because I could see the enormous effort Philip was trying to make. It seemed to me that Philip's mental state had improved through the use of regular medication, but that he had gained weight and now chain smoked. His diabetes, a side effect of the medication he was on, was also exacerbated by the large amount of sugar he still consumed.

When Mum told Philip about Dad's death, he barely nodded. He showed no emotion and shed no tears; it didn't seem to impact upon him at all. Philip asked Mum again if Dad had died - as if he was double-checking matters - but still he showed no real interest or emotion. I can't say I was surprised because I always knew he would react like this. There was no point in him going to Dad's funeral as he wouldn't really have understood what was going on and, anyway, he didn't ask to go.

Four years later Philip died. He had a mild heart attack at the care home and was rushed to Homerton Hospital in Hackney for emergency treatment. Mum and Alan went to the hospital to be with him. It was midnight when Alan texted me to let me know what was happening. I asked if they wanted me there and Alan said, 'Yes - it may be the last time we see Philip'. He was lying there on a bed, his chest festooned with an array of wires and monitoring pads. As I was getting ready to leave, I got another text off Alan saying, 'Hold off - wait till the morning'. This upset me but Alan assured me that there was little we could do at that point. Mum and Alan kept a bedside watch on Philip but then he had a massive second heart attack. The nursing staff were keeping him alive on the life support machine but his brain was dead. Though traumatised and in shock, Mum and Alan had to discuss what to do with the supervising doctors. Mum was resistant but in the end it was Alan who made the decision - switch off the life support.

Philip died on the 10th October 1999. A post-mortem was carried out and it was confirmed that Philip had died of heart failure caused by heavy smoking and by being overweight, which was compounded by the medication he'd taken over the years.

Today, Alan vividly remembers that night when the machine had to be switched off. He says he feels no remorse, only a great sense of relief that Mum's long ordeal was over. There was no chance of Philip's life being saved as he was confirmed brain dead. I cannot imagine how Alan felt having to decide to switch off the machine, but I would have agreed with him if I'd been there. I understand for sure that it's a difficult thing to decide. He was brave, I don't think I would have had the guts to do it.

Philip's death was a tragic and untimely end. I don't think it was something he expected and we all found the shock difficult to come to terms with. Given the nature of his death, we felt the funeral would be subdued and that few family or friends would attend. It was a quiet affair and Mum hid her sorrow, not wanting to show her feelings or shed tears at the sight of Philip's coffin. Her head lowered, she linked her arm heavily with mine as she watched the coffin being laid on the altar. I believe that later and in private, Mum was inconsolable.

What to say? We all went home feeling very, very sad after the funeral. There was no point having a wake because as a family we felt it was irrelevant. We wanted to have a quiet day without any hassle.

Soon afterwards, I suppose it was inevitable, I started to reminisce about the past with Philip. Many memories came flooding back, the time we'd spent together, holidays and weekends by the seaside, the fun we'd had together, the life he had lived. It haunted me for days. I also felt a dreadful remorse that I had not found a way to deal with his illness when it had become a problem. The guilt has racked me ever since. Should I have helped Philip more with his mental state? Should I have sought professional help? Or asked people who'd had experience of dealing with mental health? Had my family done enough to help Philip? My way has always been to mind my own business unless I'm asked to intervene, but I now wonder if that was enough. Reflecting on Philip's life, my mother had done so much for him by caring and trying to meet his needs. But had I?

Philip's death certainly contributed to me making decisions about certain areas of my personal life. I realised you never know what is around the corner and it made me focus on what was and is important to me. Although it 14 years since he died, his death still influences my life and what I do. Sometimes I regret my negative feelings for him, showing my hatred towards him for his actions. I really only realised afterwards that Philip was mentally ill and that his mind, body and life were absorbed, consumed, with his dreadful illness.

It was tough for Mum. She rarely talked about Philip afterwards, although she knew that he was now in a better place. When death happens suddenly and without explanation there is no easy way to deal with it. Mum loved Philip very dearly and once admitted he'd been her favourite son. Whilst she hadn't been particularly demonstrative at the funeral, her face revealed her sadness. I think all those years of nurturing Philip, and then going through all of the suffering we'd had to endure, made Mum and I both mentally and emotionally strong. We knew that life goes on.

There is a part of me that is relieved that Philip is no longer in this world. Not because of my fear and the hatred I had for him, but because I did love him in a sisterly way. The relief is mostly because I didn't want to see Philip going through all of the suffering that his illness brought upon him. I just wish he'd had a better quality of life and I could then be happy for him. It is such a tragedy that he got caught up in a web of drugs and mental illness.

The last 15 years of Philip's life at the care home were dramatically different to the previous 14 years at home. He had a dedicated key worker, money, clothes, a few treasured possessions and a room to call his own. He was given choices and encouraged to be as independent as possible. He seemed to flourish on his own. He spent time re-learning some of the basic skills of everyday life and got involved in a range of leisure activities; he enjoyed learning to cook, going to the pub for a meal, going for a drink and shopping. My Mum once asked him if he remembered being admitted to St Clements Hospital. He said, 'I remember it' and then became quiet for a couple of minutes. He then went onto say, 'I don't like it and I prefer to be here at home'. The care home had become a real home for Philip. It was heart-rending to see Philip say this but at long last he seemed to be happy. I am thankful to all the professional healthcare workers and carers who looked after him and helped him with his recovery. I met them at the funeral and they were all genuine and caring people. They commented on how difficult Philip was at the beginning but that once he was settled in, he became quite likeable.

It's difficult for me to know what Philip truly experienced in care, but I think I can take a view and that's what I'm doing here. I wonder what he would be like if he was living a 'normal' life today? I can't quite imagine him without a mental illness. Maybe he would be just an ordinary brother like any other, leading his own life. Memories of him will always live within my heart and my family. We have not forgotten him and that's why I've written this book...this work is for Philip and I dedicate my endeavour to him.

15

Mental Health and Deafness – The Stigma

Think about it. Everyone is 'mental'. Everyone is able to think about what is happening around them and the things they do. Naturally we are all emotional in different ways; we can be happy, sad, excited, bored, stressed or mad.

We're human beings and we're story tellers. To be a person is to have a story with so many things to say, so many pictures to paint. Most of us have a rich collection of experiences to relate - whether happy or sad - as there are so many challenges we have to face in this world. We have beliefs, ideas, worries and dreams about all the things we can do and more. Relationships affect us - whether that's being in love or the joys of friendship. All of this stems from how we feel, our well-being, our mental well-being. But sometimes life can be difficult for us and when it goes wrong, the effects show.

How do you explain the stigma around mental health and how it affects people's lives? Naturally, it isolates them and so people who suffer from mental illness find it difficult to relate to others what they are experiencing and how they feel. This is because they fear people's reactions and when problems are disclosed, misunderstandings can occur. Family members, friends, neighbours, work colleagues and healthcare professionals alike can fail to grasp the true intricacies of mental illness.

My own research shows that psychiatric patients are four times more likely than the average person not to have a close friend and more than a third have no one to turn to for help. They often feel that family and friends neglect them because of their illness. Families, on the other hand, can feel embarrassed when they learn that a family member is mentally ill and they usually react with a mix of shock and horror. Sometimes they will then avoid the person in question which the leads to further isolation and low self-esteem.

When my female friends visited our family home, Philip would try and make conversation with them but they were terrified of his appearance. They said that he would ask strange questions and he would come across as not making any sense. I was frequently asked how I put up with him every day but to me the answer was simple: 'Philip is my brother and the family have a responsibility to care for him'. We were, of course, embarrassed and I found that people's comments hurt. My friends would keep their visits brief as they felt very uncomfortable around Philip and struggled to cope with his outbursts. Sometimes we would go to my bedroom or the private lounge so that we could get away and be more relaxed.

The stigma of mental health has far and wide-ranging impacts. It prevents a person from going about their daily activities like shopping, going to the pub, holidays, socialising or family life. Some people have even been refused personal insurance which makes it harder for them to travel or own property. Legal complexities make it very difficult for a schizophrenic to own property even if the house or flat concerned has been inherited.

I certainly believe that people can't get jobs because of the stigma of mental health. Philip had work at one point but he was sent home because of his auditory hallucinations. His employers were fearful and reluctant to keep him on. Dad tried to persuade them to keep him, but in the end they had to let him go because they couldn't manage him.

Deaf people with mental health problems really do struggle to get work with more than a third reporting that they have been sacked or forced to resign because of their illness, whereas many never even apply for work because they know they will face painful discrimination. The stigma of Deaf people with mental health problems tends to be greater because they are labelled by both their disability and their illness. To try and escape this labelling, it has not been unknown for some Deaf people to deny their illness and to blame their behaviour on other people or medication.

I've had experience of three of my Deaf friends being admitted to the National Deaf Services, a service for Deaf people with mental health problems. All three were suffering from varying degrees of mental illness. One of them was very dear to me and was embarrassed to see me working there. I explained that as a nurse I had a role to perform and a job to do. My friendship with her was a completely different matter. It was difficult at the beginning to convince my friend that this was the case. However, with some reassurance and an explanation of the bounds of professional confidentiality, we got on very well. I confess that I was very upset to see my friend admitted and I hoped a speedy path to recovery could be determined. Certainly for me, it did feel difficult at the beginning but I drew strength from the Nursing & Midwifery Code of Conduct. I was able to keep my friend's confidence and temper her embarrassment, knowing that the Deaf community is very small and that someone, somewhere, always knows your business. I learnt that I gained a lot of respect from our patients because I always worked to maintain my professionalism and confidentiality. My friend and I go back a long way and so we would meet up for lunch once a week. I saw no reason why this should change just because she suddenly had an illness. So we'd continue to lunch and even today, we still meet up for a coffee and a chat. I don't look at my friend as an out-patient but rather as a real friend, talking about all things we like with our usual girlish ridicule and humour. Once or twice my friend has asked for informal advice about her illness and I've been more than happy to help.

When people first experience mental health problems they will often be in denial because they feel ashamed and they have no idea how or who to contact for help. If a crisis has started to develop they may contact their general practitioner for help but there are many people who don't do this and therefore receive no treatment and care.

I remember when I was a second-year student nurse at the University of Salford. We were in a class with our lecturer discussing the stigma of mental health. We talked about media interest in the famous boxer, Frank Bruno, who suffered from severe depression and was separated from his wife. The newspapers labelled Frank 'loony' and 'bonkers Bruno', printing all sorts of hurtful remarks. Frank was very upset but remained adamant that the illness could affect anybody. His best friend Harry Carpenter, the boxing commentator, was there for him throughout his illness. Frank was praised for being honest and open when people approached him and he gained a lot of support which was positive for him.

There are also other celebrities who experienced the challenges of mental illness. I read with interest of the actress Marilyn Monroe in her autobiography *Norma Jean*. Her mother Gladys was mentally unstable and financially unable to care for her when she was young, so she placed her with foster parents. Marilyn was traumatised by her mother's behavioural problems when she was a very young girl and it affected her moods. Later on she was to be blighted by depression and checked into a mental institution in 1962.

Another celebrity in the media who has spoken openly about her illness is Catherine Zeta-Jones, who suffers from bi-polar affective disorder, otherwise known as manic depression. It was not surprising to learn that, with the pressure brought on by her husband Michael's throat cancer, she was admitted to a mental health clinic in America. Many people commented on how brave she was to publically acknowledge her illness, whilst also applauding the greater awareness she had generated.

Another actress, Suzanne Shaw, related on the morning TV programme *Daybreak* how she had suffered from postnatal depression and described how she felt when she gave birth to her child. This was surprising given that ten years ago, mental illness was seen as a taboo and few people would ever think of disclosing that they were suffering from a mental illness. This goes to demonstrate that several celebrities have disclosed their illnesses and in doing so, have benefited from considerable public support.

I was also impressed that the *Coronation Street* actor Jenny McAlpine, who played Fiz Battersby, was very supportive of the mental health charity, Mood Swings. An award-winning charity based in Manchester, it was founded in 1999 to help people recover from mood problems and the severe emotional distress they can cause. Mood problems can range from periods of severe anxiety or depression to episodes of high and low mood. The effects on education, employment, family life and relationships can be devastating. The work of the charity is based on a belief that people can recover from severe mood problems and move on to lead happier and fuller lives.

Another new organisation which is making a big difference is called Time to Change. This charity has produced banners, postcards and posters with celebrities such as Ruby Wax, Stephen Fry, Patsy Palmer and Alastair Campbell, all of whom have openly admitted their mental illnesses. Ruby Wax said. 'One in five people have dandruff yet one in four people have mental health problems. I've had both'. The courageous Stephen Fry said, 'One in four people, like me, have a mental health problem. Many more people have a problem with that'.

I certainly believe Stephen Fry has been most brave in speaking of his mental illness. He has been expansive about his bipolar affective disorder and has urged other people to help him remove the stigma, shame and hidden pain the illness brings. He has made a number of television documentaries where he candidly discusses his depression and breakdowns. It seems that he copes well and is well supported by his friends. People deal with their illnesses in different ways and I was interested to hear the actress Patsy Palmer say that her 'most challenging role was hiding depression from people'. Famously, the political aide Alastair Campbell once observed that he had said to Tony Blair, 'You do know about my breakdown, don't you?'

One of the Time to Change postcards reads, 'Myth: Mental health problems are very rare. Fact: Mental health problems affect 1 in 4 people'. It goes on to comment, 'What you can do to help end discrimination: stay in someone's life and be there. If someone talks to you: listen. How do you support them: by not defining people by their mental health problems. Think about how hurtful it can be when someone calls you 'nutter', 'crazy' or 'psycho'.

One issue is that popular films such as *The Beautiful Mind*, *Donnie Darko*, and *Rain Man* reinforce the stereotypes and myths that abound around mental illness. One that captivates me, however, is *One Flew Over the Cuckoo's Nest*. I find it fascinating when I watch this film and would watch it again and again. The discrimination it portrays is harrowing to watch at times.

Time to Change aims to put an end to mental health discrimination and I find this organisation excellent at promoting the issues to people who have no understanding of the subject. The stigma will always go on but it can certainly be reduced if mental health awareness is promoted. To contact Time to Change visit www.time-to-change.org.uk

One challenge for people with mental illnesses is their treatment and recovery. Recovery can be difficult if people with mental health problems do not seek help early. It is worth encouraging people who are not aware of different mental health charities to seek them out and to get their support with the recovery process.

I attended a four-day course entitled Recovery and Social Inclusion in 2010. I found this course to be fantastic and it was a definite learning curve for me. The course was designed to introduce ideas about recovery, social inclusion and ways of helping people with their recovery journey. The course consisted of teaching about experiences, telling stories, insight and knowledge of the mental health field.

Over the four days I learnt that telling stories can help patients to move on and gain a better sense of who they are. Teachers, parents, friends or doctors all have a different version of the patients' lives. But the patients' version of what has happened to them helps us to understand their lives better. When things are difficult for patients, some like to keep a diary. This allows them to note their feelings and to also analyse what has happened to them, giving them the space to think through all that has gone on. Some prefer to draw pictures to express their feelings. When pictures are drawn by patients, the images and thoughts in their minds are often projected into artwork which can sometimes reveal the depth of their illness as well as experiences they remember from their past.

Recovery is described by people who have suffered from mental illness as a personal and unique process of changing one's attitudes, feelings, values and skills. It is a path to lead to a more satisfying and hopeful life for them even if it has limitations. Many people find that when they become mentally ill it can be devastating. Too often they feel that their life is over and that they will never be able to get better. They also feel their dreams and ambitions will not be achieved. It does not have to end like that. Listening to other patients' stories can be a source of hope and inspiration for them, even if they share this with families or friends it helps to build trust. Recovery is possible and lives can be rebuilt.

It is important for the individual to identify and think about the dreams they want to achieve and to have ambitions. We all need to have something we want to strive for and achieve. When people are not well they go into a negative spiral and say that they can't do what in fact they are capable of or that they don't have the will to do something - yet through supportive recovery they are able to lead a positive life.

Springfield Hospital in south west London has recently set up a Recovery College. It is the UK's first mental health recovery study and training facility. The College provides a range of courses and resources for service users, families, friends, carers and healthcare professionals. It also aims to support people to become experts on their own self care and to have a better understanding of mental health issues. The courses are run by mental health professionals and peers that have experience of working with and managing mental health difficulties. The College can be contacted through Springfield Hospital and it provides a wide range of information on recovery pathways.

16

Facts about Schizophrenia

T he Oxford Textbook of Psychiatry describes two basic types of schizophrenia - acute schizophrenia and chronic schizophrenia. The distinctive features of acute schizophrenia are delusions, hallucinations and interference with thinking. These are called 'positive' symptoms. The features of chronic schizophrenia are apathy, lack of drive, slowness and social withdrawal. These are called 'negative' symptoms. It is possible that a schizophrenic patient may have both negative and positive symptoms.

Emil Kraepelin (1855-1926) was the German psychiatrist who had the idea of grouping together schizophrenia and manic depression symptoms. He categorised the illness into four types, which are: catatonic (which is characterised by persons who retain a fixed and sometimes bizarre position for long periods of time without moving or talking); hebephrenic (which is characterised by having flat or inappropriate emotions, disorganised behaviour, bizarre movements and grimaces); paranoid (which is characterised by hallucinations, false beliefs); and simple (which consists of various types that do not match the criteria of the other three types). Kahlbaum was one of the first psychiatrists to discover and diagnose catatonia in 1863 and Hecker did the same for hebephrenia in 1871.

Schizophrenia is caused by an imbalance in the level of chemicals (called neurotransmitters) in the brain. These chemicals are involved in transmitting impulses through the nerves in the brain and they tend to work at junctions between nerve fibres (called synapses). When a person becomes psychotic, the balance of neurotransmitters in the brain is dysfunctional.

A person normally shows the first signs of schizophrenia in adolescence or young adulthood. This is possibly due to changes brought on by puberty. The effects of the illness are confusing and often upsetting to families and friends; it can cause a great deal of distress. People with schizophrenia suffer from difficulties in their thought processes which lead to hallucinations, delusions, disordered thinking such as flights of ideas, elated and grandiose thoughts, and unusual speech or behaviour. People affected with these symptoms find it difficult to interact with others and may withdraw from society.

People with schizophrenia clearly suffer great disruption to their lives. Families and relatives, friends and carers are also deeply affected, not just because of the distress of seeing the effects of the condition, but also the difficulties associated with providing support. When supporting someone and coping with the symptoms of schizophrenia it can be difficult for family members who remember how active or lively a person was before they became ill.

Schizophrenia is a complicated illness, which is thought to occur because of a number of different factors acting together. These factors seem to include genetic influences and trauma to the brain which may have occurred during birth. Other factors are the effects of stressful life events, and the use of illegal drugs such as cannabis. Social isolation is another factor. Each of these factors is believed to increase the risk that a person may develop symptoms.

One in 100 people will develop schizophrenia in their lifetime. Schizophrenia is found all over the world, and rates of illness are very similar from country to country. Schizophrenia is the single most destructive disease to young people. From research, it has been shown that men and women are at equal risk of developing the illness. Most males become ill between 16 and 25 years old, and females tend to develop symptoms at a later age between ages 25 and 30.

If a person is experiencing symptoms of schizophrenia, a psychiatrist, doctor or a mental health team worker is the advisable person to approach to seek professional help. It is important that family members, relatives or friends are able to seek help if a person develops schizophrenia. Ready and early intervention is critical if a successful recovery is to occur.

Treating schizophrenia with medication can help reduce and control the distressing symptoms of the illness. Some schizophrenics may discontinue treatment because of unpleasant side effects or because they become paranoid that the medication is causing them to be ill or to gain weight. In some instances the person may be influenced by other patients saying that the medication is poisonous or bad for them. Even when treatment is effective, some people find it difficult to regain the life they had previously and require other forms of help. Schizophrenics who are on long-term medication should continue to take the medication since it has a protective effect against future relapses and they should not be encouraged or persuaded to cease their prescription. Whilst medication can help control the disorder, it invariably can't cure it. But certainly regular medication helps to prevent the symptoms returning.

When I was a healthcare assistant at National Deaf Services I had a discussion with a colleague who was saying that my brother's schizophrenia must have come from someone in my family. He said that there must be mental illness in my genes. I strongly disagreed with him, saying that it was not always the case and that there were other contributing factors other than genetics - like drugs or the environment. I argued that my family had no history of mental illness or schizophrenia. Initially, I was very upset by my colleague's comments and after thinking things over for a long time, I decided to do some investigating of my own. I checked with my immediate family and asked about previous generations but there was no evidence of any mental illness. I assured my colleague that during the early years of our life, Philip did not suffer from excessive anxiety or bad behaviour. It is almost certain that Philip developed schizophrenia through his drug use. This influenced me to do more research on schizophrenia on the internet, in books, newspapers and magazines, so I do have a sense of how the illness was caused and why. There's lots of information in the public domain about schizophrenia and people do want to know what this illness is and how it is caused. Suffice to say, it's good for people to have some knowledge and understanding of what schizophrenia means and how it can affect other people's lives.

My own research has shown that schizophrenia can be either genetically passed on by the family or triggered by the environment. There are also possible environmental causes of schizophrenia. These could include a viral infection when the baby is developing in the womb, malnutrition of the mother during pregnancy or birth, or being raised in a rough and difficult environment. And as I've noted before, schizophrenia can be triggered by drugs misuse. Cannabis can cause psychotic symptoms which are worsened if the person is already mentally unwell.

Most schizophrenics can lead stable lives in the community. I am sure that from reading newspapers, listening to the news, or TV, many people assume that people with schizophrenia are all unpredictable and dangerous. The reality is that nine out of ten people with schizophrenia do not hurt themselves or others. But when schizophrenics are involved in serious incidents, the media has a field day with them. Most people who have no knowledge of mental health hear only about the violent incidents. There are all sorts of reasons why schizophrenics can become frightened or violent towards others and their outbursts are commonly directed at families and carers. It is rare for schizophrenics to assault random people in public.

Hallucinations are common in schizophrenia but can occur in other mental illness too. A hallucination happens when you hear, see, feel or smell something but actually there isn't anything there. Hallucinogenic voices may talk to you directly or they may talk to each other. It can be pleasant, rude, irritable or abusive. Some schizophrenics have described visual hallucinations as being of shadows or ghost-like figures.

I've found it fascinating working as a nurse and caring for in-patients. Every in-patient is different and their illnesses can be individually complex and challenging to manage. For many, the depth of their illness depends upon how they are affected by auditory or visual hallucinations.

One of the most interesting experiences I have known was of one young male in-patient who was admitted to Old Church, an open unit for Deaf in-patients and out-patients with a range of mental illnesses, because of his visual hallucinations and his deteriorating mental state. He described seeing different kinds of animals running across the room. He was very disturbed by the movements, frequently turning his head to follow wherever they went. On one occasion he told me that he could see tigers running fast across the wall and a herd of elephants heading towards a river. I have never come across any other patients who have described these kinds of animal hallucinations.

Most patients I have spoken to say they are communicating with other people, talking to televisions or seeing other people talking. One patient claimed to be royalty and said that he frequently visits the Queen for tea. He explained that he will soon receive millions of pounds because he is well known in society. This kind of delusion is called 'grandiose elation'.

On another occasion I remember a young male schizophrenic was admitted to Old Church for the first time. He was from a Muslim family and was quite simply terrified. He was very restless and his family were at a loss to know how they could help him. One of our nurses had developed some expertise from a psycho-intervention course which is very useful in helping families who are trying to understand mental illness. After a number of sessions with the nurse, the family began to understand why and how their son had become mentally ill. Whilst it wasn't easy, they came to terms with matters and finally accepted his illness.

Recently, we had an incident when a female schizophrenic became very distressed when reading the Metro newspaper. She approached me and showed me a picture of the deceased Michael Jackson and an article describing the different medications he had taken. One of the tablets was Lorazepam which is a drug used for its sedative, anxiety-relieving and muscle-relaxing effects. The patient was worried that because she was taking Lorazepam she would die like Michael Jackson. I explained to her that this was highly unlikely and I had to spend quite some time going through her medication to reassure her all was well.

17

My Own Journey

During my adolescent years, I always dreamed of becoming a nurse but thought it would be impossible because of my disability and the stigma that Deafness holds in the workplace. As you may well know, years ago nobody would have thought Deaf people could pursue a career in nursing. No disrespect to those Deaf people in the community but the majority are employed as manual workers and very few achieve professional status. This lack of professional achievement is a direct result of years of oppression leading to a mindset that Deaf people could not achieve, or even set out to achieve what hearing people take for granted.

During the last year at school, everyone met with the careers officer to discuss future job options they wanted to pursue on leaving. I remember meeting my careers officer and discussing my future; she asked me what I would like to do when I left school, and I replied I would like to be a nurse. She was astonished and said to me, 'You can't be a nurse; you are Deaf and you wouldn't be able to hear what's going on around you in a ward'. The careers officer filled me with no confidence at all, leaving me in tears about my job prospects. It took a long time to establish which careers were perceived as being suitable for me and eventually, with much encouragement from my teacher, I applied for a civil service job, my main reason being that as public sector employee, working for a government department or government agency, I would be entitled to an excellent pension scheme. Exactly what a girl of 15 dreams of...

It was not until the 1990s that the breakthrough came for Deaf people wanting to pursue a career in nursing. After many years of pressure from both the Deaf and hearing community - and with great support from within the nursing community - the English National Board for Nursing, Midwifery and Health Visiting finally announced that there would be a course enabling Deaf people to qualify as nursing professionals. When I found out this out, I remember thinking how great it was for the many Deaf people who wished to enter the profession and for the many who could now realise their dream of nursing.

But back to the civil service - after leaving school, I worked for the Department of Education and Science, as a specialist typist in the typing pool. I had a lot of support from my supervisor because I was just 16 years of age and obviously very new to working in an 'adult' environment. My skills developed over the years and I eventually became a desktop publisher and payroll officer. At the time of my redundancy in 1997, I had accumulated some 24 years of service.

When I began as a specialist typist in 1972, Margaret Thatcher was the then-Minister of Education and I saw her almost daily as she worked on the floor above me. She was always busy with meetings and from what I saw was nearly always surrounded by male politicians and accompanied by her chief secretary. I admired Mrs Thatcher's stamina and strong will; she never seemed fazed by the other politicians. She went on to become the UK's first female Prime Minister with a strong, powerful, personality and equally strong political views. It was her achievement and hers alone that enabled her to break through the glass ceiling of this traditionally male-dominated world. Mrs Thatcher proved that women could be leaders and has influenced many female leaders since. But that said, she was hugely divisive and most unpopular at times. Her proposal to replace the rates system with the 'Poll Tax' provoked great outrage.

After time, the Department of Education and Science announced the possibility of redundancies and invited those who were interested to consider taking voluntary redundancy. I considered this and accepted as I already had a feeling that there was no future prospect for me in civil service, especially as the Department of Education and Science was merging with the Department of Employment. The resultant organisation was called the Department of Education and Employment. I was certainly glad to have the opportunity of taking redundancy because now that I knew it was now possible for a Deaf person to qualify as a nurse, I wanted to pursue my desired career in the field of mental health nursing.

After leaving the civil service, I immediately went to the job centre to 'sign on'. I must admit I hated going there because I felt uncomfortable having to tell the claims officer what I'd being doing all day as I worked through the multitude of forms. It took about six months to find a job, six tedious months of filling in copious forms at the dole office.

In 1997, I became an auxiliary nurse and worked in the Deaf unit of the Grosvenor Nursing Agency at Springfield Hospital. I worked there for three years and this was the start of my learning curve - where I was to gain my founding experience in caring for patients with mental health issues.

But before I could commit to training as a mental health nurse, I felt that I needed to do some much-needed travelling and after discussing this with my friend Judy, I agreed that we would go backpacking around India and Nepal for five months.

The experience was incredible: the people, the culture and of course the beautiful and historical architecture that uniquely defines each country.

The Lonely Planet travellers' guide turned out to be a really useful resource. It is considered by many to be the 'bible' for Indian travel and it didn't take us long to see why. It gives detailed information on history, restaurants and interesting places to see. It also contains photographic displays of Indian culture and famous landmarks, along with maps of India and many of its cities. Without this book, we wouldn't have known how best to make the most of our adventure.

For me the most awesome place to see in India was the Taj Mahal in Agra (Uttar Pradesh state). A magnificent building which was built in 1631 by the Mughal emporer Shah Jahan in memory of his favourite wife, Mumtaz Mahal, it is considered to be an exemplary and beautiful representation of Mughal architecture, a style that combines elements from both Arabic and Indian architectural styles. It took the emperor 22 years to complete and is listed as one of the Seven Wonders of the World. Although the building was (and still is) pure white, I will never forget how its appearance changed in the fading light of dusk. The pure reflection of bright white became a romantic pink in just a few hours, emanating a feeling of true Utopia.

I remember I was feeling homesick one time when I was in Lucknow, on the eastern side of India. It was early one morning and I was sitting outside a cafe, waiting for breakfast, watching the traffic and the people passing by. I felt a sudden overwhelming feeling of nostalgia; the crowded street bustling with people going to work reminded me of London. I thought about my family, friends, work colleagues and all the people I knew back home. It had come to a point where I had the time and space to explore my own thoughts and feelings and although it was hard to be away from home, it gave me the opportunity to reflect on my past.

Among many other recollections, I started to think about my brother and how he suffered with mental illness. During that time of reflection, I came to realise that his illness was not his fault and I felt myself coming to terms with this and with the anger I had been holding on to. More crucially, I began to forgive him for some of the things he had done in the past. I almost re-scheduled my flight home to an earlier date but changed my mind. Looking back, I realise now that being in India was a turning point for me; it helped me shape how I felt towards my brother and how I felt about myself. I was able to form answers to all the questions I had posed to myself for so long. I felt stronger and somehow more independent. I was able to place a reflective distance between me, as I am now, and the 'me' that grew up over the years with my brother.

Judy and I continued our journey from India into Nepal as planned. The most memorable experience in Nepal was boarding a flight on a small charter plane from Kathmandu and flying around the Himalayas and the Sagarmatha National Park (where Mount Everest is located). Sagarmatha is the highest national park in the world, with the entire park located above 3,000m (9,700ft). It has three peaks that are higher than 8,000m, including Mount Everest. The view of the park from the plane was breathtaking; its terrain has been cut and carved by deep rivers and glaciers over millions of years, making the landscape rugged and very steep.

Returning from India and Nepal to home was a complete culture shock. I was surprised by just how beautiful the countryside in England was, covered in lush green pasture and with lovely winding roads. The roads were smooth and the traffic flow easier than in India. It felt strange to be able to drink the water straight from the tap after having to drink bottled water. It was nice to see families and friends again after so long and to be able to share my experiences. I realised that it wasn't till I returned from my travels that I was able to appreciate the many luxuries and comforts that we so easily take for granted. My memories of India and Nepal will be ones I will cherish, an inspiring journey that, indeed, shaped me forever.

With my feet firmly back on the ground in England, I decided it was time to commit to my new career.

In March 2000, I began working as a health care assistant at Old Church, National Deaf Services in Balham, London, an open unit for Deaf patients with various mental health conditions. The job involved manual handling, cleaning, building therapeutic relationships with in-patients, escorting to hospital appointments, communication support and assisting the qualified nurses with their daily duties. I used this time to learn and develop my skills, watching the experienced carers and nurses carefully!

I recall a qualified nurse observing my work and telling me that I had a natural talent for looking after patients and that she recognised that I was able to communicate clearly with them. Some of the staff found it hard, but being Deaf, I had a natural insight into the patients' cultural and linguistic backgrounds. This recognition also made me aware of just how much my approach to work had been shaped by my experience of growing up with my brother. Schizophrenia and mental illness held no secrets for me - these were conditions I had already become accustomed to.

My nursing colleagues were impressed with my skills and I was encouraged to enrol for a nursing qualification. This would lead to me becoming one of the few qualified Deaf nurses in Britain. But before I could enrol on a degree level course, I had to attend Croydon College to do an Access to Nursing BTEC course. This was because my three CSEs were not enough for entry to the degree course. I passed the access course and in September 2002, I moved up north to study at the University of Salford, Manchester.

I was one of three Deaf students in a class of about 15 hearing students. We were provided with two British Sign Language interpreters and a note taker so that we could access the lectures. Our lecturer was Naomi Sharples who was also my personal tutor. Naomi established the University's Deaf Project 2000 and worked tirelessly to recruit and champion Deaf students to become nurses. She had a good understanding of Deaf culture, having worked as a registered mental health nurse at the John Denmark Unit, Manchester, which caters for Deaf in-patients.

Deaf people's access to the nursing education project has been a part of Naomi's drive and working life since 2000. She now works for the University of Salford as the Director of Nursing in Mental Health and Learning Disability Nursing. Yet despite these responsibilities, she still remains a personal tutor to Deaf and hearing student nurses.

In 2000, she was awarded a commendation in the Nursing Standard Awards, Mental Health category, for her hard work in this area. Her tireless endeavours have also been commended by the European Society for Mental health and Deafness at the highest level with the World Health Organisation.

In my first year at University I was admittedly a little homesick. My new accommodation comprised of a basic bedsit in a student block of flats, which was quite different to the two-bedroom house in Bromley that I was used to. Somehow I managed to sail through the course. Having the support of other students, my friends and the 12-week study placement at the Old Church National Deaf Services all helped. It was strange to have left my placement as a health care assistant and to return, on completion of my studies, as a student nurse. My new role was obviously quite different, but slowly and over time, I began think of myself as a student nurse.

From September 2002-2005 I studied on the Diploma in Nursing (Mental Health) and following successful completion

I became a registered mental health nurse. I felt overwhelmed when I qualified and was immensely proud of myself! I had achieved what I had set out to gain. I will always remember the quote from the Nursing & Midwifery Council: 'Great nurses teach, but also inspire'. This quote has served as my motto and encouragement throughout my career.

I have since learnt that all of the 14 Deaf students who enrolled at the University of Salford achieved their Diplomas. Recently, two went on to study for the Advanced Standing Diploma, showing that they could progress to a higher level alongside their hearing peers. Until recently, the University of Salford was the only university that encouraged Deaf students to apply for nursing courses. Their success rate for Deaf students has averaged 90% - a remarkable achievement!

Most of the Deaf nurses who became registered mental health nurses have gone on to find work within the Deaf mental health field, be it in forensic services such as Rampton or Alpha Hospitals or within more generic services such as the National Deaf Services at Old Church, London, or the John Denmark Unit in Manchester. A few, however, left the profession and used the Diploma as a stepping stone to pursue other career interests.

In October 2005, I went for an interview for the post of staff nurse on the Connaught Ward at Rampton Hospital. I was incredibly nervous and left the interview thinking I had come across poorly, that there was no way they would offer me the job. Yet the very next day I received an e-mail offering me the job. After a tiresome wait of three months, I completed the hospital's induction course and eventually started work at Rampton in January 2006.

I worked there for three years and found it a real challenge. Situated near Retford in Nottinghamshire, it's one of three maximum security hospitals in England and Wales offering treatment to offenders with mental disorders. The other two maximum security hospitals are Broadmoor and Ashworth.

Rampton Hospital is divided into four areas of provision: Mental Health, Learning Disabilities, Personality Disorder and Women's Services.

At Rampton, the Connaught Ward differed from the other wards in that it housed the Deaf Service, accommodating up to 10 Deaf male patients who have a range of mental illnesses, personality disorders and learning disabilities. The patients were placed according to their communication needs and the culturally appropriate environment they required - rather than according to their specific diagnosis. Their communication skills varied from those who had native fluency in British Sign Language through to those who had minimal sign language skills and communicated through the use of pictures and gestures. Because of their personality disorders, the male patients were not easy to communicate with and many had suffered childhood abuse or neglect, which often leads to emotional problems. Patients with personality disorders are very difficult to treat because the diagnosis covers such a broad range of symptoms and because some cannot be treated with medication. Many of them spend many years going through rehabilitation therapy and attending therapy groups. These therapy groups comprise a number of courses focusing on specific areas such as emotional and social skills and art therapy along with specific support with alcohol, drugs or other substance misuse.

In 2008, I was the co-facilitator of two therapeutic groups, the Alcohol & Drugs Substance Misuse Group and the Social Skills Group. The challenge was to address the psychological, spiritual and social needs of patients and to meet those needs at the patients' own levels, working with them on an agreed path to recovery. Some patients are quick to learn the benefits of rehabilitation and engage well in sessions. But some do not. It takes a lot of time and patience to teach patients to understand the aims of the programmes and the therapy within. My co-facilitator and I used a lot of simple English and drew on a flipchart to visually describe and demonstrate the meanings of different topics we were working on.

As a nurse, my primary role and aim were to care for patients. I was the only qualified Deaf nurse on the Connaught Ward and the first Deaf person to be employed as a nurse by Rampton Hospital. All the other qualified nurses and nursing assistants were hearing. Some of them had NVQ Level 1 and 2 BSL skills and one team leader had achieved NVQ Level 4 in BSL. At times I used BSL interpreters to facilitate access to meetings, support my training and supervision, assist with ward rounds and for making final adjustments to my written English.

Understandably, as a maximum security hospital, Rampton had very strict security procedures and relied on staff being in VHF radio contact with the control room to gain information on patients' whereabouts. For example, if patients had woodwork lessons, they had to be escorted with staff to the woodwork area and the control room had to be informed. Subsequently, when the patients had finished their lessons and they had to be escorted back to their ward, the control room was once again informed.

It wasn't easy being the only Deaf nurse working at Rampton. There was a lot to deal with, especially working with people who had a limited understanding of Deaf culture and issues. Whilst there were two Deaf support workers on the ward who occasionally taught basic sign language skills, and although Deaf awareness training was readily available, some of the staff just simply couldn't be bothered. To make things even more difficult, a number of the staff couldn't get used to working with Deaf people, let alone alongside a Deaf qualified nurse, so for me there were challenges all around.

I worked at Rampton Hospital for three years and the job challenged me in ways I would never have imagined. No two days were the same, no day predictable, and I always came away having learned something new about myself and other people.

Many people have asked me how it was that I could work there supporting patients who are criminals. I would explain that it was difficult at first, but that I had to think of myself as a professional nurse whose role is to support and treat patients. There are many offenders who experience problems with mental health, substance abuse or have personality disorders and quite a number of them have been excluded from healthcare. Most of these individuals have a poor lifestyle, have grown up in poverty and neglect and have offended in later life. I discussed the lack of consistent treatment with some of the patients at Rampton, including those who experienced years of drug and alcohol abuse, and found some of their stories to be just shocking. I did find it particularly hard developing a therapeutic relationship with patients who were sex offenders but after a while I got used to it. Some people said I must have been brave to work at Rampton Hospital but it was a good opportunity for me to acquire forensic knowledge and to become familiar with working in a maximum security environment.

My nursing experience at Rampton included liaising with the security staff to ensure that patients are safe within the hospital grounds. About 90% of the patients at Rampton were detained under Section 37/41 of the Mental Health Act, meaning that instead of sending the offender to prison, the Crown Court decided that the person would benefit from being admitted to a hospital where they would receive treatment for their specific mental health problem. This decision may also have been taken because of concerns about public safety. The Secretary of State at the Home Office decides when the patient can be given leave, so long as all agreed conditions have been complied with.

In December 2008, I completed NVQ Level 4 in British Sign Language (BSL) and in March 2009 I was promoted to work as a clinical nurse co-ordinator (band 6) at Old Church, Balham, which is part of the National Deaf Services, south west London and St George's NHS - quite a mouthful! I was delighted and proud when I became a nurse, but was even more proud to be appointed into my current band 6 role. An achievement which was, dare I say, far beyond most people's expectations of me. Despite the barriers I've faced, I have always pushed myself to achieve and to utilise all the training opportunities presented to me. I enjoy the challenges that life brings and my busy workload always keeps me on the go. My co-ordinator role requires me to manage both staff nurses and health care assistants, and ensure the ward works in good order. There are still more skills in management - theory and practice - I can learn from the ward and I believe that this is something I am doing every day. The ward manager always supports me in my role and is readily available to advise and help me. With this support I hope to further develop my management skills, to enhance evidence-based practice in nursing, and to promote the work of nursing at the National Deaf Services.

The Deaf Services is a specialist mental health service for the management, support and treatment of mentally ill Deaf patients whose first language is British Sign Language. The staff group working at the Deaf Services features Deaf and hearing professionals who sign. Old Church is a multi-function building housing an in-patients unit with 15 beds, a specialist Deaf community mental health team, a Specialist Assertive Outreach team, a psychology team, a psychotherapy team, a speech and language therapist, a social worker, an occupational therapist, a dedicated administrative team, medical and nursing teams and a sign language interpreter team. It is quite an enterprise and in October 2012, the whole set-up moved to a new ward at Springfield Hospital as part of a regeneration initiative.

The qualified nurses are either registered mental health nurses or learning disability nurses. Staff are rotated over a 24-hour period, seven-days-a-week shift pattern. They work with a range of Deaf patients who are admitted for various issues;

these vary from mental illnesses, emotional issues, neurological deficits, forensic histories and challenging behavioural and personality disorders, through to obsessive compulsive disorders, alcohol and substance misuses. Deaf patients who have been diagnosed with autism are also admitted.

Initially, I have to admit that I had no knowledge about people with autism and how to deal with them. Yet, after a few years of seeing these patients, I began to recognise their symptoms and to see how they cope with the challenges of communication. Autism is a lifelong brain disorder that is normally diagnosed in early childhood. People with autism have difficulties in communicating and in forming relationships with others. They find it hard to make sense of the busy world around them. Patients who have autism and Deafness (a dual diagnosis) can be very hard to care for. People with autism usually have unusual patterns of language development and frequently exhibit no eye contact. They have very narrow interests and engage in repetitive and sometimes challenging behaviours.

Some patients with learning disabilities lack the ability to make decisions for themselves and struggle to make informed decisions. This is why the Mental Capacity Act 2005 is used for their protection. This legislation aims to support people with learning disabilities and sets out the principles that should be followed by care staff engaged in caring for them. Patients with learning disabilities can therefore work with staff to make decisions through the use of simple language and visual aids. An assessment of mental capacity is usually carried out to determine whether an individual has the capacity to make a decision on their own or whether support is needed. A staff nurse or doctor is usually responsible for the best interests of the patient and any important decisions will be made in consultation with the patients' families and carers.

The unit takes patients subject to the requirements of the Mental Health Act and/or the Mental Capacity Act and also accepts patients who have been admitted informally. It requires two approved mental health practitioners to section a patient. Dependent on the mental state of the patient, both have to agree that admittance to a secure setting would be beneficial for the patient and also in the public interest.

Clearly there are great sensitivities around mental illness. This is understandable and this is why I sought the advice and support of Psychiatrist Dr Helen Miller. Helen has been hugely supportive and has encouraged me no end, giving me permission to publish this story.

When I look back to the start in life that my education did *not* give me, and the journey I have travelled since, I am not only proud of my achievements but I also want to tell the world: 'Deaf people CAN do it!' And, indeed, I'm looking forward to the day when Deaf staff nurses are commonplace.

Conclusion

For me, writing this book has been most therapeutic. It has encouraged me to think and reflect on my life. It has been a very emotional experience and not an easy task. I have had to think, revise and review again throughout the chapters.

I was really surprised when I finally came to the end. I thought I would have writer's block and not be able to finish, but the thought of Philip's illness has inspired me.

Recently I had a deep conversation with my friend Hannah about mental and emotional issues. We discussed this book and I explained some of the stories to her and how I felt during that time. She was fascinated to hear about Philip and how he affected my family and friends and also my ambition to become a qualified nurse. She told me that people knew what I'd been through and were supportive; that I was admired by healthcare professionals within the mental health field and how many had commented on the quality of my work.

Some of my friends said that Philip's illness may have affected me mentally or emotionally. I certainly admit to being insecure, such as not being able to trust easily and I sometimes have hard times, feeling emotionally low. I am sure a lot of people have similar feelings and most of us go through those emotions at some point in our lives.

I was reminded by the people who have close contact with me that this book would be a rare story because I am Deaf myself and I am writing about a Deaf schizophrenic brother. Who else has lived this story and had the experience of this situation?

It is not easy to live with a schizophrenic at home or in the public. A schizophrenic can be the most complex person to look after. I realised that Philip had been living with us for about 13 years before he was first diagnosed and up until then had received no treatment. I often think about my parents who fought tooth and nail to look after Philip and I am ever so grateful that they stayed together to support not only themselves, but the whole family. My parents suffered enough throughout the years, nursing Philip and coping with so many of the problems he generated. I honestly thought they would give up and walk away but they didn't.

I have been really lucky and fortunate with my family. They have filled me with love and given me a deep sense of satisfaction.

Thinking about theories and practice and how other nurses have become famous, I have read with interest about a certain nurse called Dr Hildegard Peplau. She is known as the mother of psychiatric nursing because she has influenced different areas of nursing. Dr Peplau originally introduced the concept of the nurse/patient relationship in the 1940s when patients did not actively participate in their care. It was her idea to develop the nurse/patient relationship and to be more aware of the patients' needs. Dr Peplau's theories and clinical work also developed the field of psychiatric nursing. She wrote a book called *Interpersonal Relations in Nursing* in 1952, from which I would like to quote:

'Somewhere, somehow, at some time in the past, courageous nurses determined these skills, learned them, fought for the right to use them, refined them, and taught them to other nurses.'

Dr Peplau has inspired me to think of theories relating to nurse/patient relationships. Nurses here at Deaf Services, Springfield Hospital have very therapeutic relationships with patients and I admire them for their proactive and hard work. I am proud to say that we all have excellent clinical skills and are specialised in the complexities of Deafness and Deaf issues associated with mental health, including myself.

Within the Deaf community I have been asked to give mental health awareness presentations and have done so, giving examples from my life experience. I find this very rewarding. People ask questions after the presentations and a lot of them are unaware of the reality of mental health and illness. They usually find that they learn some interesting new things about schizophrenia. Some people have positive and negative views on schizophrenia but, as I explain to them, it is important for them to be aware of mental health issues.

Every day I live with the emotional and mental scars of my past, but they remind me just how far I have come and how, no matter what happens, there is no going back. I know I have moved on and life is different now; I have a contented life with family and special friends whom I love dearly. They share my world. I spend my time reaching out to others who find themselves in the dark throes of despair. I want people to know that however good or bad things are, there is always a way through - I am living proof of this. I have lived with a schizophrenic brother and struggled at times - but I got through it.

It has taken a while to turn my collective memories into this volume. I started writing in 2009. I've come a long way and it's been hard work. But the rewards for me have been immense. Through the darkness and despair, I think I've now unravelled the signs.

Useful References

Mackenzie clan - *www.clan-mackenzie.org.uk/clan/history*

Robert Burns - haggis, tatties and neeps - *Scottish-at-heart.com (2011)*

Arbroath smokies - *http://www.bbc.co.uk/food/recipes/search?keywords=Arbroath+smokies (2008)*

The National Health Service 1948 – *Wikipedia (2010)*

The 'Model Traffic Area', Downhills Park – *Wikipedia (2011)*

Decibels/defining hearing loss - www.hear-it.org.uk *(2011)*

Jewish immigrants - *Wikipedia (2008)*

A guide to electro-convulsive therapy (also known as ECT) - *www.bbc.co.uk/health/electro_convulsive_therapy.shtml*

Mental Health and Deafness - *Peter Hindley and Nick Kitson (2000)*

One in One Hundred Schizophrenia - *www.oneinonehundred.co.uk (2008)*

Schizophrenia - *www.rcpsych.ac.uk/mentalhealthinformation/mentalhealthproblems/Schizophrenia.co.uk (2008)*

Shorter Oxford Textbook of Psychiatry - *Michael Gelder, Richard Mayou and Philip Cowen (2001 Oxford University Press)*

Dr Hildegard Peplau - *Wikipedia, the encyclopaedia (2011)*

actionDEAFNESSBooks

Are you interested in deaf issues? Want to learn sign language? If so, check out our fabulous online store! Action Deafness Books is one of the UK's leading online retailers of deaf-related resources including books and dvds. We pride ourselves on competitive prices and excellent customer service and are constantly sourcing fresh literary talent and exciting new products.

We are delighted to have published works by accomplished deaf authors such as Nick Sturley (*Innocents of Oppression*) and Stuart R Harrison (*Same Spirit Different Team: The Politicisation of the Deaflympics*), thus empowering deaf authors and enabling them to showcase their talents. Other works we have published include the fascinating *Unravelling the Signs: My Life with a Deaf Schizophrenic Brother* by Sylvia Kenneth and the moving *Meanwhile I Keep Dancing* by Tamsin Coates.

Books like these, together with our popular sign language resources, promote deaf awareness throughout the wider community, allowing our customers to expand their knowledge and experience the rich and beautiful culture of deaf people. Our aim is to spread the word - literally!

We are proud to have worked with renowned authors such as Jacqueline Wilson (Tracy Beaker novels), Julia Donaldson (The Gruffalo) and Joyce Dunbar (the Mouse & Mole series) and have championed their works at various literary events and via our social media channels.

Contact us at: adbooks@actiondeafness.org.uk
Visit: www.actiondeafnessbooks.org.uk
Follow us on Twitter: @ActionDeafBooks
Facebook: www.facebook.com/actiondeafnessbooks